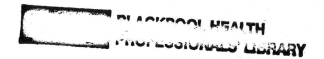
GET THROUGH MRCP
PART 1: 1000 MCQs AND
BEST OF FIVES

By

Una Coal

MD FRCSEd F

Editorial A
Eric Beck F

British Library Cataloguing in Publication Data
A catalogue record for this book is available from the British Library

ISBN: 1-85315-526-8

Phototypeset by Phoenix Photosetting, Chatham, Kent
Printed by Bell & Bain Ltd, Glasgow

Preface

From May 2002, the MRCP (UK) Examination has been completely reformatted and implemented. This book is designed to prepare prospective candidates for the new MRCP Part 1 examination. I am very pleased to be collaborating with Dr Eric Beck, an examiner with the Royal College of Physicians and has participated in the construction of the new MRCP examination.

The new MRCP Part 1 (UK) Examination now consists of 60 true/false multiple choice questions and 100 'best of fives' (BOFs). Negative marking has now been replaced by a zero mark for each Don't Know or Nil response. A select number of pre-test questions will be introduced into Parts 1 and 2, however these scores will not be counted. Criterion referencing will be employed to mark Papers 1 and 2. This means that each question has a predetermined level of difficulty with a corresponding estimate of the percentage of candidates who are expected to get a particular question correct. The pass mark is then adjusted accordingly. The pass rate for Part 1 in future may, therefore, vary from the previous fixed 35% of all candidates. This book covers Part 1 and presents a total of 1000 MCQs and BOFs or 6 complete exams with bonus MCQs. The emphasis is on topics stressed in the MRCP examination. Answers are cross-checked with the Oxford Textbook of Medicine as referenced by the Royal College of Physicians.

Una Coales
July 2002

I would like to dedicate this book to Professor John M. Porter MD

Contents

Preface — iii
Dedication — iv
Recommended Texts and References — vi
Introduction — 1

MRCP Paper One Multiple Choice Questions (MCQs) — 4
Answers to Paper One MCQs — 15
MRCP Paper One Best of Fives (BOFs) — 20
Answers to Paper One BOFs — 48
MRCP Paper Two MCQs — 55
Answers to Paper Two MCQs — 66
MRCP Paper Two BOFs — 71
Answers to Paper Two BOFs — 95
MRCP Paper Three MCQs — 102
Answers to Paper Three MCQs — 113
MRCP Paper Three BOFs — 119
Answers to Paper Three BOFs — 143
MRCP Paper Four MCQs — 150
Answers to Paper Four MCQs — 162
MRCP Paper Four BOFs — 167
Answers to Paper Four BOFs — 189
MRCP Paper Five MCQs — 196
Answers to Paper Five MCQs — 208
MRCP Paper Five BOFs — 214
Answers to Paper Five BOFs — 240
MRCP Paper Six MCQs — 247
Answers to Paper Six MCQs — 259
MRCP Paper Six BOFs — 265
Answers to Paper Six BOFs — 292
Bonus MCQs — 299
Answers to Bonus MCQS — 307

Recommended texts and references

American Psychiatric Association (2000) *Diagnostic and Statistic Manual of Mental Disorders*, 4th edn. American Psychiatric Association, Washington D.C.

Collier J.A.B. *et al.* (1994) *Oxford Handbook of Clinical Specialties*, 3rd edn. Oxford University Press, Oxford.

Fauci A. *et al.* (1997) *Harrison's Principles of Internal Medicine*, 14th edn. McGraw-Hill, New York.

Fitzpatrick T.B. *et al.* (1990) *Color Atlas and Synopsis of Clinical Dermatology*, McGraw-Hill, New York.

Ganong W.F. (1993) *Review of Medical Physiology*, 16th edn. Appleton & Lange, Connecticut.

Hope R.A. *et al.* (1998) *Oxford Handbook of Clinical Medicine*, 4th edn. Oxford University Press, Oxford.

Jawetz E. *et al.* (1987) *Review of Medical Microbiology*, 17th edn. Appleton & Lange, Connecticut.

Jenkins R *et al.* (2000) *WHO Guide to Mental Health in Primary Care*, The Royal Society of Medicine Press, London.

Kumar P.J. *et al.* (1998) *Clinical Medicine*, 4th edn. Baillière Tindall, London.

McMinn R.M.H. (1990) *Last's Anatomy Regional and Applied*, 8th edn. Churchill Livingstone, London.

MRCP (UK) Part 1 Examining Board (1999) *MRCPUK Part 1 Papers 1997/98*, Royal College of Physicians, London.

Paterson C.R. (1987) *Essentials of Human Biochemistry*, Churchill Livingstone, London.

Royal Pharmaceutical Society of Great Britain (2001) *British National Formulary*. British Medical Association, London.

Rubenstein D. *et al.* (1991) *Lecture Notes on Clinical Medicine*, 4th edn. Blackwell Science Publications, Oxford.

The Editorial Board (2001) *Advanced Life Support Course Provider Manual*, Resuscitation Council (UK), London.

Tomb, D.A. (1999) *Psychiatry*, 6th edn. Lippincott, Williams and Wilkins, Baltimore.

Website of MRCP(UK) Central Office provides up to date information: http//www.mrcpuk.org

INTRODUCTION

THE NEW MRCP (UK) EXAMINATION 2002 sees the completion the implementation of the recommendations made in the major review of the examination in 1997.

The changes relating to the **PART ONE** examination are:

Part 1 syllabus:
First published by the MRCP (UK) Central Office in November 1999 and to be regularly updated.

Two papers:
MCQ PAPER ONE (as before)

60 STEMS each with 5 answers giving 300 TRUE / FALSE (300 marks)

MCQ PAPER TWO (new)

100 STEMS each with 5 answers from which ONLY ONE is selected giving 100 TRUE (100 marks)

Negative marking
An incorrectly selected answer will no longer be given a negative mark (−1). This guessing is no longer penalised.

Criterion referencing
The difficulty of each question will be assessed by a panel of experts and a notional score agreed. The sum of the ease and difficulty of questions will determine the **PASS MARK** for that paper and all candidates achieving it will pass. So the easier the paper the higher the pass mark and vice versa.

This book incorporates all the changes in the new **PART ONE** examination and will help you prepare for it by providing:

6 complete **PART ONE** papers each comprising 60 TRUE/ FALSE (T/F) MCQs and 100 BEST OF FIVE (BOF) MCQs. The composition of each paper will follow the **CONTENT** and **SEQUENTIAL ORDER** questions as in the actual examination but not quite so rigidly.

The 360 T/F and 600 BOFs will cover a substantial part of the syllabus. The same topics, but in a different format, may occur in more than one paper occasionally, as in the actual examination; for example, a particular stem might generate three separate sets of questions on investigation, diagnosis and treatment. If these were to appear as three consecutive questions in one paper, they could be so inter-related as to cue the candidates to the correct answer for all three or, conversely, an incorrect answer to the first might falsely cue the other two.

The **ANSWER KEY** to the questions is annotated to explain some of the more difficult answers. Each question will be **CRITERION REFERENCED** using a three point scale of how difficult or easy a candidate just passing the whole examination would find that particular question:

*   25–50%   "just passing" candidates expected to get correct
* *   50–75%   "just passing" candidates expected to get correct
* * * 75–100%   "just passing" candidates expected to get correct.

The overall profile of the make up of each paper can then be translated into a NOTIONAL pass mark for each paper (**this is purely a guide for the candidate and may differ from the method of calculation in the actual examination**).

You will see that the pass mark in the **SIX** 60 T/F MCQ papers ranges from 204 to 228 marks out of a possible 300 marks (68 to 76%) which is higher than in past examinations. This largely reflects the abolition of negative marking which will inevitably raise the scores obtained.

The pass mark in the new six 100 BOF MCQ papers ranges between 76 and 78 out of a possible 100 marks. Remember you are required to select **ONE** completion only in each BOF and there is **ONE** mark for the correct answer; as is implied in the appellation BOF the four distracter completions should be plausible partly correct answers but attract no marks.

Advice on answering MCQs

However childish it may sound the first advice given to examination candidates in their school days still holds good:

READ THE QUESTION CAREFULLY BEFORE ANSWERING IT.

Question setters try very hard to avoid ambiguity in the terms they use and candidates should be aware of the meaning of frequently used wordings:

CHARACTERISTIC: if not present would make you unsure of the diagnosis
RECOGNISED: does happen but may be uncommon
MOST/MAJORITY: over 50%
CAN/MAY: a correct answer
ALWAYS/NEVER: usually an incorrect answer as medicine, like life, rarely has certainties; setters usually therefore avoid these words
LONG ANSWERS: often tend to be correct – but not always.

Look out, particularly in BOFs, for questions requiring ONE NEGATIVE answer e.g. "all the following are correct except".

Setters try to avoid bias in the completions in a T/F paper by ensuring that the number of true and false completions are roughly equal (150 **TRUE** and 150 **FALSE** overall in a 60 T/F MCQ PAPER).

Likewise the ordering of completions A to E is increasingly in alphabetical order unless it upsets the sense of the question.

Make sure you are familiar with the system of transcribing your answers into the boxes on the mark sheet. Use the 2B pencil provided and rub out thoroughly any you consider on review, to have entered incorrectly.

With the abolition of negative marking there is now an incentive against leaving answers blank or marking the sheet **DON'T KNOW** box earning no mark; so make a guess at **TRUE** or **FALSE** and try and answer each BOF.

When selecting the best of five in a BOF rather than weighing each answer against the other four see if you can decide what you would have given as the best answer unprompted and check whether it appears amongst the five offered – you are more likely to be right. This format can however mean that the best answer sometimes will not be listed if it is obviously so superior to all the others (which would turn the question into a best of one!)

MRCP Paper One MCQs

Questions

1. Immediate effects following spinal cord hemisection include

   A loss of contralateral touch sensation
   B spinal shock
   C ipsilateral spastic paralysis
   D contralateral flaccid paralysis
   E impairment of ipsilateral proprioceptive impulses

2. Which of the following statements regarding surface anatomy are correct?

   A The middle meningeal artery is located behind the pterion.
   B The left lobe of the liver extends into the 5th intercostal space.
   C The spleen is normally palpable.
   D The neck of the pancreas is at the tip of the 9th costal cartilage.
   E The bifurcation of the aorta is just below the umbilicus.

3. Erythropoietin

   A is synthesised in the liver
   B is raised in polycythaemia rubra vera
   C may be raised in cerebellar haemangioblastoma
   D is raised by living in high altitude
   E is metabolised in the kidney

4. Features associated with a meningomyelocoele include

   A hydrocephalus
   B congenital dislocation of the hips
   C congenital heart disease
   D urinary incontinence
   E paraplegia

5. Autosomal dominant inherited conditions include

   A achondroplasia
   B dystophia myotonica
   C cystinosis (Fanconi Syndrome)
   D idiopathic haemochromatosis
   E osteogenesis imperfecta

6. Chorionic villus sampling

   A is offered at an earlier gestation date than amniocentesis
   B may diagnose maternal rubella
   C is associated with a higher abortion rate than amniocentesis
   D is indicated for HIV positive mothers
   E is a recognised screening test for Down's Syndrome

7. The following antibiotics are teratogenic

   A metronidazole
   B amoxycillin
   C ciprofloxacin
   D erythromycin
   E trimethoprim

8. Hepatitis B is associated with

   A infection with a RNA virus
   B Hepatitis D
   C an incubation period of up to 12 months
   D low infectivity if HbeAg is present
   E carrier status if HbsAg is present for >3 months

9. Insects are vectors of the following diseases

   A Lyme disease (Borrelia burgdorferi)
   B Weil's disease (Leptospirosis icterohaemorrhagica)
   C yellow fever
   D trypanosomiasis (sleeping sickness)
   E leishmaniasis

10. Epstein–Barr virus is the cause of or trigger for

   A Bell's palsy
   B Burkitt's lymphoma
   C Hodgkin's lymphoma
   D nasopharyngeal carcinoma
   E Crohn's disease

11. The following are nucleoside reverse transcriptase inhibitors used for the treatment of HIV infection

   A abacavir
   B nelfinavir
   C nevirapine
   D retrovir
   E ritonavir

12. The following antibiotics are bacteriocidal

   A amoxycillin
   B cefuroxime
   C chloramphenicol
   D erythromycin
   E tetracycline

13. Cutaneous manifestations of malignancy include

   A pemphigoid
   B erythema multiforme
   C necrobiosis lipoidica
   D pityriasis alba
   E dermatitis herpetiformis

14. Pernicious anaemia is characterised by

   A hypersegmented neutrophilis
   B hypergastrinaemia
   C pancytopaenia
   D bone marrow hypoplasia
   E hyperbilirubinaemia

15. Risk factors for deep venous thrombosis include

   A protein S deficiency
   B antithrombin III deficiency
   C hypercholesterolaemia
   D lupus anticoagulant
   E alcoholic cirrhosis

16. Treatment of psoriasis includes

   A cyclosporin
   B emollients
   C topical 5-fluorouracil (FU)
   D topical steroids
   E vitamin D analogue cream

17. The following drugs are contraindicated in asthmatics

   A diclofenac
   B atenolol
   C coproxamol
   D morphine
   E doxapram

18. The following statements regarding antidiuretic hormone (ADH) are correct

   A It is synthesised in the posterior pituitary gland.
   B It decreases GFR.
   C It decreases water permeability in the distal tubules.
   D It increases with activation of baroreceptors.
   E Its action is increased by nicotine.

19. Peripheral neuropathy may be associated with the following drugs

   A nitrofurantoin
   B carbamazepine
   C isoniazid
   D thalidomide
   E pyrazinamide

20. Pulmonary oedema can be caused by

   A aspiration of pleural effusion
   B bronchiectasis
   C cerebral injury
   D high altitudes
   E mitral stenosis

21. Aortic stenosis is associated with

   A left ventricular hypertrophy
   B atrial fibrillation
   C pulmonary oedema
   D pulmonary hypertension
   E left parasternal heave

22. The following statements regarding rheumatoid arthritis (RA) are correct

   A There is an association with HLA-B27.
   B High rheumatoid factor is associated with a poor prognosis.
   C Atlanto-axial subluxation may occur with general anaesthesia.
   D Rheumatoid factor is an anti-IgM autoantibody.
   E Ulnar deviation is more pronounced in the dominant hand.

23. Causes of atrial fibrillation include

   A anxiety
   B myocardial ischaemia
   C constrictive pericarditis
   D mitral stenosis
   E hypothyroidism

24. Left atrial myxoma may be associated with

    A finger clubbing
    B pyrexia
    C sudden loss of consciousness
    D mitral valve prolapse
    E atrial fibrillation

25. Clinical features of bronchiectasis include

    A cerebral abscess
    B finger clubbing
    C halitosis
    D haemoptysis
    E nasal polyps

26. Causes of diffuse pulmonary fibrosis include

    A sarcoidosis
    B Wegener's granulomatosis
    C systemic sclerosis
    D haemosiderosis
    E cyclosporin

27. Gardner's syndrome is associated with

    A Skull osteomas
    B Hutchinson's teeth
    C pigmented ocular fundal lesions
    D dermoid tumours
    E adenomatous polyps of the colon

28. Causes of lung abscess include

    A acute osteomyelitis
    B streptococcal pneumonia
    C alcoholism
    D mycoplasma pneumonia
    E achalasia

29. Bronchial malignancy is associated with exposure to

    A chromium
    B beryllium
    C asbestos
    D aspergillus
    E coal dust

30. Clinical features of dystrophia myotonica include

A cardiomyopathy
B glucose intolerance
C progressive proximal muscle weakness
D ptosis
E tetany

31. Causes of sudden painless loss of vision include

A giant cell arteritis
B retinitis pigmentosa
C central retinal vein thrombosis
D malignant hypertension
E malignant melanoma of the choroid

32. Cerebellopontine angle tumours may cause

A contralateral facial palsy
B visual field defect
C ataxia
D unilateral sensorineural hearing loss
E tinnitus

33. Peripheral neuropathy is associated with the following conditions

A bronchial carcinoma
B vitamin B_1 deficiency
C acute renal failure
D hyperthyroidism
E rheumatoid arthritis

34. Multi-infarct dementia is associated with

A impaired concentration
B disorientation to time and place
C impaired memory retention
D depersonalisation
E a familial tendency

35. Recognised features of anorexia nervosa include

A hyperkalaemia
B sinus bradycardia
C primary amenorrhoea
D constipation
E hirsuitism

36. Dysphagia is associated with

    A pharyngeal pouch
    B cervical spondylosis
    C motor neurone disease
    D myasthenia gravis
    E sliding hiatal hernia

37. Risk factors for gastric cancer include

    A blood group O
    B pernicious anaemia
    C *Helicobacter pylori* infection
    D acanthosis nigricans
    E giant hypertrophic gastritis (Menetrier's disease)

38. Recognised features of Crohn's disease include

    A nail clubbing
    B renal oxalate stones
    C acute pancreatitis
    D uveitis
    E large-joint polyarthritis

39. Recognised associations of ulcerative colitis include

    A ischiorectal abscess
    B ankylosing spondylitis
    C hepatitis
    D amyloidosis
    E sclerosing cholangitis

40. Irritable bowel syndrome is associated with

    A heartburn
    B greater prevalence in females
    C abdominal colic relieved by bowel opening
    D rectal mucus
    E weight loss

41. Good points to note in critical reading appraisals are

    A use of randomised control trials
    B data with narrow confidence intervals
    C a P value of less than 0.5
    D use of case-control studies for small numbers of subjects
    E methods documenting selection criteria of subjects

42. Central periumbilical abdominal pain features in the following conditions

A acute appendicitis
B occlusion of the superior mesenteric artery
C sickle-cell trait
D acute pancreatitis
E acute cholecystitis

43. Idiopathic haemochromatosis may be associated with

A chondrocalcinosis
B diabetes mellitus
C heart failure
D loss of libido
E steatorrhoea

44. Aims in the management of diabetes mellitus include

A an albumin creatinine ratio (ACR) of <3.5 in a male and <2.5 in a female
B explaining that one cigarette for a diabetic is the equivalent of three cigarettes in a non-diabetic
C a cholesterol level of <2.5 mmol/l in the elderly
D check HbA1C annually
E a systolic BP of <140 in the elderly

45. Porphyria cutanea tarda is associated with

A an increase in activity of hepatic uroporphyrinogen decarboxylase
B underproduction of uroporphyrins
C hepatitis C as a trigger factor
D haemochromatosis
E linear skin eruptions

46. The following statements regarding antidiuretic hormone are correct

A It is synthesised in the posterior pituitary gland.
B It decreases GFR.
C It decreases water permeability in the distal tubules.
D It increases with activation of baroreceptors.
E Its action is increased by nicotine.

47. Features of osteitis deformans (Paget's disease) include

    A decreased hydroxyproline in the urine
    B deafness
    C sarcomatous changes
    D osteoporosis circumscripta
    E high calcium and phosphate levels

48. The following statements regarding rheumatoid arthritis are correct

    A There is an association with HLA-B27.
    B High rheumatoid factor is associated with poor prognosis.
    C Atlanto-axial subluxation may occur with general anaesthesia.
    D Rheumatoid factor is an anti-IgM autoantibody.
    E Ulnar deviation is more pronounced in the dominant hand.

49. Gardner's syndrome is associated with

    A skull osteomas
    B Hutchinson's teeth
    C pigmented ocular fundal lesions
    D dermoid tumours
    E adenomatous polyps of the colon

50. The following statements regarding critical reading are correct

    A The introduction of a paper should include the design of the
      experiment.
    B The results should include the drop-outs.
    C The discussion should include the applicability.
    D The methods should discuss outcome measures.
    E The paper should declare any conflicts of interest.

51. Polycystic ovarian disease is associated with

    A increased risk of breast carcinoma
    B serum FSH greater than LH during the first week of the cycle
    C increased serum sex hormone binding globulin
    D secondary amenorrhoea
    E increased levels of serum androstenedione

52. Osteoporosis is a recognised complication of

    A ovarian dysgenesis
    B short-term heparin usage
    C primary biliary cirrhosis
    D hypothyroidism
    E Addison's disease

53. The following diseases and test findings are correctly paired

A gout – positively birefringent crystals in synovial fluid joint puncture
B multiple sclerosis – monoclonal protein band on electrophoresis
C SLE – low serum complement
D Paget's disease – raised serum alkaline phosphatase
E rheumatic fever – raised antistreptolysin-O titre

54. Acute renal failure is associated with

A hypokalaemia
B hypernatraemia
C hypercalcaemia
D polycythaemia
E increased urinary sodium excretion

55. Favourable points to note in critical reading appraisals are

A use of randomised control trials
B data with wide confidence intervals
C a P value of less than 0.5
D use of case-control studies for small numbers of subjects
E methods documenting selection criteria of subjects

56. The following sites are recommended to be swabbed for gonorrhoea detection in a female

A urethra
B high vagina
C endocervix
D rectum
E low vagina

57. Agents that cause phytophotodermatitis include

A parsnip
B celery .
C giant hogweed
D cow parsley
E poison ivy

58. Malignant melanoma

A has a better prognosis if the growth phase is radial as opposed to vertical
B is treated by block dissection
C may be treated with high dose interferon
D staging is by sentinel node biopsy
E has a better prognosis if it occurs on the back

59. Erythema nodosum may be associated with

    A BCG vaccination
    B Lyme disease (*Borrelia burgdorferi*)
    C *Helicobacter pylori*
    D sarcoidosis
    E leprosy

60. Retinal detachment

    A is less common in myopic eyes
    B may present with field defects
    C may present with sudden visual flashes of light
    D is a hazard of the sport of bungee jumping
    E can occur due to melanoma

Criterion Referencing Marks

* – 25–50% of candidates expected to get correct
** – 50–75% of candidates expected to get correct
*** – 75–100% of candidates expected to get correct

The notional PASS MARK is 216/300 or 72%

1. TTTFT **

2. TTFTT ***

3. FFTTF ** Erythropoetin is produced in the kidney and metabolised in the liver. Production is raised in secondary polycythaemia.

4. TTTTT **

5. TTFFT ** cystinosis (Fanconi syndrome) is an autosomal recessive condition. Other autosomal dominant inherited conditions include neurofibromatosis, adult polycystic disease of the kidneys, familial adenomatous polyposis and Huntington's chorea.

6. TFTFF * CVS has a higher abortion rate than amniocentesis (<1%). Chorionic fetal tissue is sent for DNA analysis and gene probing. Results may be obtained in 48 hours. CVS is a diagnostic test and not a screening test for Down's.

7. FFTFT **

8. FTFFF *** Hepatitis B is infection with a DNA virus. It is associated with an incubation period of up to 6 months, high infectivity if the HbeAg is present and carrier status if the HbsAg is present for >6 months.

9. TFTTT **

10. FTTTF **

11. TFFTF * Nelfinavir and ritonavir are protease inhibitors. Nevirapine is a non-nucleoside reverse transcriptase inhibitor (NNRTI).

12. TTFFF ***

13. FFFFF *** Cutaneous manifestations of malignancy include dermatomyositis, thrombophlebitis migricans (cancer of the pancreas), and acanthosis nigricans.

14. TTTFT ***

15. TTFTF *** Risk factors for DVT include general anaesthesia, immobilisation, combined oral contraceptive pill, protein C and S deficiencies, lupus anticoagulant, antithrombin III deficiency, trauma, malignancy, varicose veins, and smoking, which increases plasma fibrinogen levels.

16. TTFTT *** Topical 5-FU is recognised treatment for actinic keratosis.

17. TTFTT *** Asthma is exacerbated by beta-blockers and by NSAIDs.

18. FTFFT ** ADH is synthesised in the hypothalamus. It increases water permeability in the collecting tubules.

19. TFTTF **

20. TFTTT **

21. TFTFF *** Aortic stenosis is characterised by a basal systolic murmur. A left parasternal heave is associated with pulmonary stenosis.

22. FTTFT ** RA is associated with HLA-DRW4 and not HLA-B27. Rheumatoid factor is anti-IgG autoantibody.

23. FTTTF *** Hyperthyroidism may cause atrial fibrillation.

24. TTTFF **

25. TTTTF ***

26. TFTFF*** Cyclophosphamide and not cyclosporin is associated with diffuse pulmonary fibrosis.

27. TFTTT ** Hutchinson's teeth are a sign of congenital syphilis.

28. TFTFT *** Lung abscess is usually caused by a staphylococcal pneumonia not a streptococcus.

29. TFTFF ** Coal dust is associated with coal worker's pneumoconiosis.

30. FTFTF ** This condition causes progressive distal muscle weakness and hypogonadism.

31. TFTTF *

32. FFTTT **

33. TTFFT *** Peripheral neuropathy is associated with chronic renal failure not acute and hypothyroidism (carpal tunnel syndrome) and not hyperthyroidism.

34. TTTTF ***

35. FTTTF *** Anorexia nervosa is associated with hypokalaemia and lanugo hair.

36. TFTTF ***

37. FTTTF *** Blood group A is associated with an increased risk of gastric carcinoma.

38. TTFTF *** Crohn's disease is also associated with amyloidosis, aphthous ulceration, cholelithiasis, cigarette smoking, delayed puberty, episcleritis, large-joint monoarthritis, and pyoderma gangrenosum.

39. FTTTT *** Ulcerative colitis is also associated with uveitis and pyoderma gangrenosum.

40. FTTTF ***

41. TTFTT ** A P value of less than 0.05 is desirable and indicates statistical significance in clinical research.

42. TTFFF *** Sickle cell anaemia may present with central abdominal pain.

43. TTTTF ***

44. FTTFT ** The aim is for an ACR <3.5 in a female and <2.5 in a male as men have a higher creatinine value due to more muscle mass. The ideal HbA1C should be <7% and should be monitored every 3 to 6 months.

45. FFTTF * Porphyria cutanea tarda is associated with a decrease in activity of hepatic URO-D and an overproduction of uroporphyrins.

46. FTFFT *** ADH is synthesised in the hypothalamus. It increases water permeability in the collecting tubules.

47. FTTTF ** There is an increase in urinary hydroxyproline. Calcium and phosphate levels are normal.

48. FTTFT ** Rheumatoid arthritis is associated with HLA-DRW4 and not HLA-B27. Rheumatoid factor is an anti-IgG autoantibody.

49. TFTTT *** Hutchinson's teeth is a sign of congenital syphilis.

50. FTTTT ** The design of an experiment should be mentioned under methods and not in the introduction. The introduction should mention the background and aim of the study.

51. FFFTT ** Polycystic ovarian disease is associated with an increase in LH/FSH ratio and a decrease in serum SHBG. PCO is also associated with an increased risk of endometrial carcinoma.

52. TFTFF ** Osteoporosis may be a complication of long-term heparin therapy or thyrotoxicosis.

53. FFTTT *** Pseudogout is associated with positively birefringent crystals. Multiple myeloma is associated with a monoclonal protein band on electrophoresis.

54. FFFFF *** Acute renal failure is associated with hyperkalaemia, hyponatraemia and hypocalcaemia.

55. TFFTT ** A P value of less than 0.05 is desirable and indicates statistical significance in clinical research.

56. TFTTF *

57. TTTTF * Phytophotodermatitis is caused by the chomophore furocoumarins (plants) and causes linear skin eruptions 1–2 days post-exposure to the plant and UVA. Poison ivy results in contact dermatitis.

58. FTTTF ** Melanoma occurring in the BANS areas (back, arm, neck and scalp) are associated with a worse prognosis, stage for stage.

59. TFFTT *** Erythema nodosum is also associated with infections with chlamydia, yersinia, tuberculosis, and streptococcus.

60. FTTTT *** Retinal detachment is more common in myopic eyes.

MRCP Paper One BOF's

In these questions candidates must select one answer only

Questions

1. A 50-year-old diabetic woman presents with fever and a dusky red erythematous eruption over the left side of her face. The MOST likely organism would be

   A *Staphylococcus aureus*
   B Group B streptococcus
   C Group A streptococcus
   D Herpes zoster virus
   E Herpes simplex virus

2. A 23-year-old woman complains of an offensive green vaginal discharge. On examination she has an inflamed cervix. The MOST useful investigation is

   A gram stain of an endocervical swab
   B wet film of a high vaginal swab
   C darkfield microscopy
   D virology on an endocervical swab
   E pH of a high vaginal swab

3. The MOST appropriate antibiotic would be

   A amoxycillin 3 gms stat
   B doxycycline 100 mg bd for 7 days
   C ciprofloxacin 500 mg as a single dose
   D metronidazole 400 mg bd for 5 days
   E clotrimazole pessary 500 mg as a single application

4. A 22-year-old HIV-positive Ugandan man presents with hypo-pigmented anaesthetic annular lesions with raised erythematous rims and painful nodules on his legs. On examination, a thickened ulnar nerve is palpated at the elbow and running into the lesions. He is also noted to have multiple transverse white lines on his fingernails. The MOST appropriate treatment would be

A standard TB treatment, discontinue the protease inhibitor and use alternative anti-retroviral drugs until the TB has been treated
B give dapsone alone
C prednisolone
D give rifampicin and dapsone
E give benzylpenicillin

5. A 17-year-old boy presents with pain on swallowing. On examination he has trismus, palatal petechiae and enlarged tonsils. His sclerae are jaundiced. The MOST likely causative organism is

A *Streptococcus pneumoniae*
B hepatitis B virus
C Epstein–Barr virus
D herpes simplex virus
E *Clostridium tetani*

6. A 36-year-old pregnant woman presents with high fever, jaundice, vomiting and drenching sweats. She had returned from Brazil a month ago. On examination she is also noted to have hepatosplenomegaly. Her test results are as follows

White cell count	11.5×10^9/L
Hb	8.0 gm/dL
Platelets	100×10^9/L
Plasma glucose	3 mmol/L
Plasma sodium	130 mmol/L
Plasma potassium	3.6 mmol/L
Plasma creatinine	180 µmol/L

The MOST useful diagnostic investigation is

A Dengue fever serology
B microscopy of thick blood film with Giemsa stain
C Mantoux test
D blood cultures
E Lassa fever serology

7. The SINGLE factor giving rise to a poorer prognosis would be

   A white cell count
   B plasma creatinine level
   C age
   D pregnancy
   E anaemia

8. Lymphatic filariasis (Wuchereria bancrofti) is associated with all of the following EXCEPT

   A blindness
   B elephantiasis
   C conjunctival loa loa
   D urticaria
   E pulmonary infiltrates

9. A 23-year-old female with Hodgkin's disease presents with small, white mucosal flecks in her mouth that can be wiped off. The MOST likely diagnosis is

   A lichen planus
   B candidiasis
   C aphthous ulcers
   D squamous cell carcinoma
   E infectious mononucleosis

10. A 20-year-old healthy man presents with acute shortness of breath, fullness in the head and blackouts. He smokes 10 cigarettes a day and drinks socially. He is noted to have a ruddy plethora, JVP 6 cm and dilatation of veins on his chest wall. Diagnosis is BEST confirmed by

   A bronchoscopy and biopsy
   B chest x-ray
   C lymph node biopsy
   D thoracic CT scan
   E bone marrow aspirate

11. A 40-year-old woman presents with fatigue, dyspnoea, and paresthesiae. On examination she has a red tongue. Her blood film shows hypersegmented neutrophils, a Hb 9 gm/dL and an MCV 120 fl. The MOST likely diagnosis is

   A vitamin B_{12} deficiency
   B iron deficiency
   C coeliac disease
   D sideroblastic anaemia
   E hypothyroidism

12. A 20-year-old woman presents with recurrent epistaxis. She admits to having heavy periods. Blood pressure is 90/60 and her pulse 100. There are bruises of different ages over her extremities but no splenomegaly. Her test results are as follows

    White cell count 8×10^9/L
    Hb   11.5 gm/dL
    Platelets 20×10^9/L
    Bleeding time   prolonged
    Antinuclear antibody negative

    The MOST likely diagnosis is

    A non-accidental injury
    B systemic lupus erythematosis
    C idiopathic thrombocytopaenia
    D thrombotic thrombocytopaenic purpura
    E sickle cell disease

13. A 40-year-old man presents with fever, sweating and weight loss. On examination he is noted to have splenomegaly. Blood test results

    White cell count 100×10^9/L with neutrophilia
    Hb   11 gm/dL
    Platelets 200×10^9/L
    Plasma uric acid   500 μmol/L (210–480)
    Plasma alkaline phosphatase   500 IU/L (30–300 IU/L)
    Serum B12   1 nmol/L (0.13–0.68 nmol/L)
    Leucocyte alkaline phosphatase low

    The MOST likely diagnosis is

    A chronic lymphocytic leukaemia
    B chronic myeloid leukaemia
    C acute myeloid leukaemia
    D acute lymphoblastic leukaemia
    E septicaemia causing leukaemoid reaction

14. The following statements regarding testicular tumours are correct EXCEPT

    A Seminomas usually present in men in their 40s.
    B Teratomas are radiosensitive.
    C Cryptorchism is a risk factor.
    D The contralateral testicle should be biopsied, if there is a history of infertility.
    E After orchidectomy the disease is staged by chest and abdominal CT scan.

15. A 30-year-old man presents with a tender swollen testicle. He states that he was hit in the groin while playing sports. On examination, the borders of the testicle are irregular, and the testicle is heavy and woody. There is no associated lymphadenopathy. He is also noted to have gynaecomastia. There are no external signs of trauma. In this age group, the MOST likely diagnosis is

A testicular torsion
B epididymo-orchitis
C seminoma
D teratoma
E testicular haematoma

16. A 70-year-old man presents with bone pain and severe gout. On examination he is noted to have a large tongue, and a tender left calf with a large non-infective necrotic ulcer. Blood test results

plasma calcium	3.9 mmol/L
alkaline phosphatase	300 IU/L (30–300 IU/L)
plasma urea	10 mmol/L
plasma creatinine	300 µmol/L
ESR	50 mm/hr

The BEST test to confirm the diagnosis is

A Serum uric acid
B bone marrow examination
C serum electrophoresis
D urine electrophoresis
E bone scan

17. A 20-year-old man back from hitchhiking through South America two weeks previously now presents with explosive, watery, foul-smelling diarrhoea and weight loss. On examination, he has abdominal distension. His stools are greasy and contain mucous. The MOST appropriate treatment would be

A ciprofloxacin
B oral prednisolone
C metronidazole
D oral rehydration
E pancreatic enzyme supplements

18. A 40-year-old woman on carbamazepine for trigeminal neuralgia now complains of severe dizziness. The drug that may have potentiated the effects of carbamazepine is

A combined oral contraceptive pill
B erythromycin
C chloramphenicol
D omeprazole
E thiazide diuretics

19. A 35-year-old indigent man is taking long-term anti-tuberculous chemotherapy. He now complains of itching and diarrhoea. He has poor memory and emotional blunting, making it difficult to understand him. The MOST likely diagnosis is

A chronic renal failure
B pellagra
C liver disease
D drug allergy
E scabies

20. An 87-year-old man is noted to have an altered level of consciousness. The serum glucose is 37 mmol/L with a serum sodium of 163 mmol/L. He has no prior history of diabetes. He has been on intravenous fluids for a week with IV cefuroxime and metronidazole for a chest infection. The MOST appropriate treatment would be

A insulin sliding scale, heparin and 0.45% normal saline
B insulin sliding scale, heparin and 0.9% saline
C insulin sliding scale, 0.9% normal saline
D insulin sliding scale, 0.45% normal saline
E insulin sliding scale, dextrose saline

21. A 40-year-old actor with insulin-dependent diabetes mellitus is started on propranolol for stage fright. He collapses on stage. He has not changed his insulin regime. His glucose is 1.5 mmol/L. The MOST beneficial advice you would offer him after treatment would be

A discontinue propranolol
B carry a chocolate bar
C decrease his humulin insulin
D decrease his actrapid insulin
E carry glucagon

22. A 50-year-old schizophrenic presents with drooling saliva and involuntary chewing movements. He walks with a shuffling gait. The MOST likely diagnosis is

A Parkinson's disease
B extrapyramidal side-effect of medication
C autonomic side-effect of medication
D anticholinergic side-effect of medication
E lithium toxicity

23. A 50-year-old farmer presents with acute shortness of breath, dizziness and severe headache. His skin is red in colour, and he smells of bitter almonds. He mentions that he had been using rodenticides. His condition rapidly deteriorates. The MOST likely agent that is poisoning him is

A cyanide
B arsenic
C organophosphate
D warfarin
E paraquat

24. A 45-year-old male psychiatric patient with long-term bipolar disorder presents with vomiting, muscle twitching and tremor. He was started on bendrofluazide recently and self-prescribes ibuprofen for headaches. Blood pressure 90/50. His gait is ataxic. He then has a series of epileptic fits. The drug MOST likely to be responsible is

A lithium
B phenothiazine
C benzodiazepine
D ecstasy (methylenedioxy methamfetamine)
E ibuprofen

25. You are on ward rounds and notice that a young patient is coughing briskly. He has just been commenced on benzylpenicillin for acute tonsillitis complicated by trismus. He states he does not know if he is allergic to any drugs. He becomes short of breath. His pulse is 110 beats/minute and he now cannot complete sentences. The MOST appropriate management for this patient would be

A administer 0.5 ml adrenaline of a 1:10,000 solution intravenously for suspected anaphylaxis

B administer 0.3 mg adrenaline intramuscularly for suspected new-onset asthma attack

C administer oxygen at 15 L/min and give nebulised salbutamol 5 mg for suspected severe asthma attack

D administer oxygen at 15 L/min and 0.5 ml adrenaline of a 1:1000 solution intramuscularly for suspected anaphylaxis

E administer oxygen at 10 L/min and give IV hydrocortisone 200 mg immediately for anaphylactic shock

26. A 20-year-old man presents with ingestion of paraquat-containing pesticide two hours prior. The MOST appropriate initial management is

A 100% oxygen and urine test to confirm paraquat absorption

B tracheal intubation

C gastric lavage followed by activated charcoal therapy and tracheal intubation

D oral administration of repeated-dose activated charcoal with magnesium sulphate every 4 hours until charcoal is seen in the stool

E haemodialysis

27. A 22-year-old man presents with fever one hour after his first injection of benzylpenicillin therapy for primary syphilis. He complains of headache, muscle pains and chills. On examination: pulse 110, respiratory rate 20/min and blood pressure 100/60. White cell count is 12.5×10^9/L with neutrophilia. The MOST likely explanation is

A Jarisch–Herxheimer reaction

B drug anaphylaxis

C neurosyphilis

D meningitis

E HIV-conversion illness

28. A 50-year-old man complains of difficulty in hearing and dyspnoea. He is noted to have a nasal septal perforation and a blood pressure of 140/90. His urinalysis shows red cells, protein and casts. The chest-x-ray reveals opacities. The MOST likely diagnosis is

    A tuberculosis
    B amyloidosis
    C Goodpasture's syndrome
    D acute tubulointerstitial nephritis
    E Wegener's granulomatosis

29. A 13-year-old girl presents with a painful and swollen knee. There is no history of trauma. A tender lump is palpated over the tibial tuberosity. The MOST likely diagnosis would be

    A osteomyelitis
    B chondromalacia patella
    C juvenile rheumatoid arthritis
    D osteosarcoma
    E apophysitis of the tibial tubercle (Osgood–Schlatter disease)

30. A 40-year-old woman complains of disabling joint pains. On examination you note scaly plaques over her anterior shins and knees. She has tried diclofenac for the arthralgia and wonders if there is any connection with the rash. The MOST useful treatment for her joints now would be

    A oral prednisolone
    B methotrexate
    C codydramol
    D topical 0.5% hydrocortisone
    E dithranol 0.1% cream

31. A 40-year-old woman complains of intolerance to cold weather and cold running water. On examination you note she has a beaked nose, radial furrowing of the lips and facial telangiectasiae. On examination of her hands you notice sausage-like digits and tapered fingers. The MOST discriminating investigation to establish her diagnosis is

    A anticentromere antinuclear antibody
    B rheumatoid factor
    C full blood count
    D chest x-ray
    E barium swallow

32. A 15-year-old girl presents with fever and red, hot, swollen wrists and knees. On examination there is a diastolic mitral murmur not heard again later during her admission and a pink ring-shaped rash with slightly raised edges on the trunk. Initial blood results show a raised ESR and leukocytosis. The MOST likely diagnosis is

A gonorrhoea infection
B systemic lupus erythematosus (SLE)
C rheumatic fever
D infective endocarditis
E juvenile rheumatoid arthritis (Still's disease)

33. A 20-year-old man presents with buttock pain radiating down both legs and heel pain. On examination he has marked kyphosis and limitation of chest expansion. ESR and CRP are raised. The MOST likely diagnosis is

A lumbar disc prolapse
B sacro-iliitis
C spondylolisthesis
D spinal stenosis
E ankylosing spondylitis

34. A 44-year-old woman complains of headaches and nosebleeds. Blood pressure is 160/100 in the right arm and 130/80 in the left arm. She complains of cold legs. The MOST likely diagnosis would be

A acromegaly
B Marfan's syndrome
C coarctation of the aorta
D Kawasaki's disease
E Takayasu's arteritis

35. A 50-year-old man presents to A and E complaining of 30 minutes of severe crushing mid-chest pains with no relief from GTN. He has a history of angina. His pulse is 105 and his BP 115/60. The 12-lead ECG shows normal sinus rhythm only. The FIRST drug to administer would be

A morphine
B oxygen
C gaviscon
D streptokinase
E atropine

36. A 40-year-old woman with a history of angina presents with severe chest pain for 30 minutes. Her pulse is 45 and her blood pressure 80/60. Her ECG shows second-degree heart block. The FIRST drug to administer would be

   A lignocaine
   B atropine
   C adrenaline
   D procainamide
   E amiodarone

37. A 40-year-old patient is brought to Casualty by ambulance in pulseless electrical activity (PEA). You are told he was given adrenaline. The NEXT step would be to

   A evaluate for reversible causes
   B defibrillate with 200J
   C administer verapamil
   D administer amiodarone
   E administer morphine

38. A 30-year-old drug addict is noted to have a pansystolic murmur heard best at the bottom of his sternum. Giant "cv" waves are present in the jugular venous pulse. The MOST likely diagnosis would be

   A ventricular septal defect
   B pulmonary regurgitation
   C pulmonary hypertension
   D tricuspid regurgitation
   E pulmonary stenosis

39. A woman in the 29th week of pregnancy collapses in a crowded casualty waiting room. She is not breathing and has no palpable pulse when seen by the SHO. The MOST appropriate initial management is

A call for help, place the patient in the supine position and commence CPR until the crash trolley arrives

B call for help, for the crash trolley and the obstetrician on call, place the patient on a trolley with a pillow under the right buttock and flank and commence CPR

C call for the crash team, obstetric and paediatric registrar on call, place the patient on a trolley with a pillow under the left buttock and flank and commence CPR until the crash trolley arrives

D call for help, place the patient on a trolley with a pillow under the right buttock and flank, and wheel the patient straight up to labour ward for an emergency Caesarian-section

E call for help – cardiac arrest and for the obstetric and paediatric registrars on call, place the patient on a trolley with a pillow under the right buttock and flank, wheel the patient into the resuscitation room, give 100% oxygen, continue CPR until the defibrillator ECG leads are attached and a rhythm confirmed

40. A 55-year-old man has been treated with three consecutive shocks of 200J, 200J and 360J for ventricular fibrillation. The morphology of his rhythm does not change. The MOST appropriate next step in management is

A administer 4th shock at 360 Joules immediately

B recheck pulse and administer 4th shock at 360 Joules

C recheck pulse and administer amiodarone 300 mg IV if the systolic BP is <90

D recheck pulse and blood pressure, commence CPR and administer lignocaine 50 mg if the systolic BP is <90

E recheck pulse and blood pressure, commence CPR and administer amiodarone 300 mg IV if the systolic BP is >90

41. A 55-year-old farmer complains of dry cough, exertional dyspnoea, joint pains and weight loss. He is noted to have finger clubbing. On x-ray there are bilateral diffuse reticulonodular shadowing at the bases. The MOST likely diagnosis is

A bronchial carcinoma

B bronchiectasis

C cryptogenic fibrosing alveolitis

D mesothelioma

E extrinsic allergic alveolitis

42. An 18-year-old known asthmatic presents with severe wheezing and a respiratory rate of 30 and a pulse of 120. She is using her accessory muscles and appears distressed. She is apyrexial. The MOST appropriate initial management would be

A IM adrenaline
B oxygen and nebulised salbutamol
C IV dexamethasone
D endotracheal intubation
E IV penicillin

43. A 25-year-old woman is brought to Casualty by ambulance having sustained gross maxillofacial deformities following a high speed RTA. She is now agitated and hypoxic despite high-concentration oxygen having been administered by face mask by the paramedics. The MOST appropriate immediate intervention is

A endotracheal intubation
B nasopharyngeal airway
C oropharyngeal airway
D cricothyroidotomy
E laryngeal mask airway

44. A 14-year-old boy with cystic fibrosis presents with pneumonia. He also suffers from mild renal failure. The MOST appropriate antibiotic treatment is

A tobramycin and carbenecillin
B ciprofloxacin
C tetracycline
D erythromycin
E cephalosporin

45. A 70-year-old alcoholic man presents with sudden onset of productive purulent cough. The chest x-ray shows consolidation of the left upper lobe. The MOST likely pathogen is

A staphylococcus aureus
B streptococcus pneumoniae
C klebsiella pneumoniae
D mycoplasma pneumoniae
E pseudomonas aeruginosa

46. A 40-year-old longstay patient in a psychiatric hospital presents with fever, abdominal pain, dry cough and worsening confusion. Blood tests reveal neutrophilia, lymphopaenia and hyponatraemia. Chest x-ray shows right-sided lobar consolidation. The MOST likely diagnosis is

A tuberculosis
B streptococcus pneumonia
C legionella pneumonia
D klebsiella pneumonia
E staphylococcus pneumonia

47. A 60-year-old dairy farmer presents with fever, cough and shortness of breath. Coarse end-inspiratory crackles are present. Chest x-ray shows bilateral fluffy nodular shadows. The MOST likely diagnosis is

A extrinsic allergic alveolitis
B aspergilloma
C cryptogenic fibrosing alveolitis
D histoplasmosis
E blastomycosis

48. A 40-year-old man presents with dry cough, exertional dyspnoea and weight loss. On examination he is noted to have finger clubbing and fine end-inspiratory crepitations are heard. Chest x-ray shows bilateral reticulonodular shadowing at the lung bases. Lung function tests show reduced lung volumes, normal FEV1 and FVC ratio but reduced individual values, and reduced transfer factor. ANA and rheumatoid factor are absent. The MOST likely diagnosis is

A extrinsic allergic alveolitis
B sarcoidosis
C lymphangiitis carcinomatosa
D cryptogenic fibrosing alveolitis
E histiocytosis X

49. A football player presents with a drop foot after receiving a kick to his right leg. He can neither dorsiflex nor evert the foot. Sensation is lost over the front and outer half of the leg and dorsum of the foot. The MOST likely diagnosis is

A superficial peroneal nerve injury
B common peroneal nerve injury
C tibial nerve injury
D lateral popliteal nerve
E sural nerve injury

50. A 50-year-old diabetic man presents with a unilateral facial nerve palsy and severe earache. On auroscopic examination, he has granulation tissue deep in the external auditory meatus. The MOST likely diagnosis is

A Bell's palsy
B sarcoidosis
C facial nerve schwannoma
D otitis externa complicated by local osteomyelitis (malignant otitis externa)
E suppurative otitis media

51. A 40-year-old man presents with progressive confusion and tremor. On examination, he has extensor plantar reflexes. The MOST useful investigation would be

A HIV serology
B computerised tomography (CT scan)
C drug screen
D Mantoux test
E VDRL

52. A 45-year-old man with a history of epilepsy presents with several weeks of fluctuating levels of consciousness. On examination his pupils are unequal. The MOST discriminating investigation is

A HIV serology
B computerised tomography (CT scan)
C electroencephalogram
D drug levels
E lumbar puncture

53. A 23-year-old woman complains of general fatigue, muscle ache and double vision. On examination you note ptosis, but the pupils are equal round and reactive. She tires easily from talking. The MOST discriminating investigation would be

A thyroid function tests
B antinuclear antibody
C smooth muscle antibody
D lumbar puncture
E anti-acetylcholine receptor antibodies

54. A 60-year-old hypertensive presents with a painful right eye. On examination he is noted to have right partial ptosis and right fixed dilated pupil. The eye is looking downwards and outwards. The MOST likely diagnosis is

A trochlear nerve palsy
B abducens nerve palsy
C incomplete oculomotor nerve palsy
D posterior communicating artery aneurysm
E optic neuritis

55. A 50-year-old man complains of stabbing pains in his chest and calves. He walks with a wide-based gait. On examination he has ptosis and small, irregular pupils. He has absent knee jerk reflexes. The MOST likely diagnosis is

A subacute combined degeneration of the cord
B syringomyelia
C tabes dorsalis
D Friedreich's ataxia
E multiple sclerosis

56. A 40-year-old man presents with numbness and tingling sensation in his feet. He is noted to have distal sensory loss and absent ankle jerk reflexes. The knee-jerk reflexes are exaggerated. He drinks heavily and smokes cigars. Blood pressure 160/90 with a pulse of 90. Full blood count reveals a macrocytic anaemia. The MOST likely diagnosis is

A syringomyelia
B tabes dorsalis
C Wernicke–Korsakoff syndrome
D vitamin B6 deficiency
E subacute combined degeneration of the cord

57. A 60-year-old man presents acutely with vertigo and vomiting. On neurological examination there is right facial numbness, an ipsilateral ataxia of arm and leg and a contralateral loss of pain and temperature sense. The MOST likely diagnosis is

A posterior cerebral artery infarction
B middle cerebral artery infarction
C anterior cerebral artery infarction
D posterior inferior cerebellar artery infarction
E vertebrobasilar ischaemia

58. A 60-year-old man presents with headache and gradual loss of central vision and loss of red/green discrimination. He is being treated with atenolol for hypertension and has just been diagnosed as having pernicious anaemia. He drinks 4 units a week and smokes 20 cigarettes a day. The MOST likely diagnosis is

A basilar migraine
B cerebral tumour
C tobacco amblyopia
D central retinal artery occlusion
E central retinal vein occlusion

59. An 80-year-old woman complains of sudden painless loss of vision in her right eye. She has facial pain on chewing. The MOST likely diagnosis is

A acute glaucoma
B retinal detachment
C cranial arteritis
D basilar migraine
E optic neuritis

60. A 25-year-old man presents to Casualty with an alkaline chemical injury to his eyes. He complains of burning eyes. On examination he has white eyes with blanched out blood vessels (limbal ischaemia). The MOST appropriate treatment would be

A apply local anaesthetic and irrigation with sterile H_2O
B test pH with litmus paper and neutralise with acid
C refer urgently to ophthamology specialist
D apply local anaesthetic and sweep the conjunctiva with a cotton bud
E place the head of the patient in a filled sink of water

61. A 40-year-old diabetic complains of seeing flashing lights and floaters in his eyes. On examination he is noted to have a unilateral irregular field defect. The MOST likely diagnosis is

A migraine with focal aura
B vitreous haemorrhage
C retinal detachment
D acute angle closure glaucoma
E central retinal artery occlusion

62. A 40-year-old woman complains of double vision, worse at night. She had a similar episode 10 years ago that resolved spontaneously. Her visual acuity is worse in the right eye and colours appear less bright. Her vital signs are normal. The MOST discriminating investigation is

    A fundoscopic examination
    B MRI scan
    C slit lamp examination
    D vitamin A levels
    E antinuclear antibodies

63. A 20-year-old heroin addict presents with weight loss, diarrhoea and confusion. On examination he has purple papules on his legs. The MOST useful investigation is

    A echocardiogram
    B blood cultures
    C HIV serology
    D chest x-ray
    E drug levels

64. A 20-year-old slightly withdrawn man states he experiences auditory hallucinations. He is noted to have poverty of speech and a flat affect. The MOST likely diagnosis would be

    A schizophrenia
    B manic-depressive disorder
    C delirium
    D dementia
    E opioid abuse

65. A 70-year-old man presents with confusion. On examination he is noted to have fixed pupils, nystagmus and an inability to look outwards. He has a broad-based gait. The MOST likely diagnosis is

    A Marchiafava–Bignami syndrome (degeneration of the corpus callosum)
    B Wernicke–Korsakoff syndrome
    C lateral medullary syndrome
    D vertebrobasilar insufficiency
    E vitamin B$_{12}$ deficiency

66. A 60-year-old alcoholic man presents with confusion and unsteadiness for several weeks. Blood pressure is 190/110 and pulse 60. His pupils are unequal and his reflexes generally brisk. The MOST likely diagnosis is

A epidural haematoma
B subdural haematoma
C subarachnoid haemorrhage
D Wernicke–Korsakoff syndrome
E viral encephalitis

67. A 45-year-old woman presents with severe itching, recent pale stools and dark urine. On examination there is darkened skin pigmentation, xanthelasma and hepatomegaly. Her test results are as follows

Serum bilirubin   15 μmol/L
Serum alkaline phosphatase   400 IU/L (30–300 IU/L)
AST   40 IU/L (5–35 IU/L)

The MOST likely diagnosis is

A sarcoidosis
B primary biliary cirrhosis
C sclerosing cholangitis
D acute cholecystitis
E common bile duct gallstones

68. A 70-year-old woman presents with progressive dysphagia and food regurgitation. On examination she has halitosis and a small lump on the left-side of her neck.

The MOST likely diagnosis is

A achalasia
B branchial cyst
C diffuse oesophageal spasm
D pharyngeal pouch
E myasthenia gravis

69. A 50-year-old man presents in shock with rigors and a temperature of 40°C. He is jaundiced and is tender on palpation of the liver, which is felt 5 cm below the costal margin. Dark concentrated urine is noted upon Foley catheter insertion. The FIRST investigation would be

A liver function tests
B blood cultures
C abdominal ultrasound
D hepatitis A, B and C virology
E endoscopic retrograde cholangiopancreatography (ERCP)

70. A 55-year-old woman complains of sudden severe central abdominal pain radiating to her back and vomiting. She prefers to sit forwards on her stretcher. Temperature is 39°C, BP 100/60 and pulse 112. On examination she has a markedly tender epigastrium and a bruise over the left flank. She has a history of gallstones. She denies smoking or alcohol. She takes HRT. The MOST discriminating investigation would be

A plain abdominal x-ray
B serum bilirubin and liver function tests
C serum amylase
D full blood count
E abdominal ultrasound

71. A 60-year-old man presents with increasing abdominal girth. On examination you elicit shifting dullness. You decide to obtain an ascitic fluid tap. The following should be routinely requested on the fluid EXCEPT

A cell count
B Gram stain and culture for bacteria and AFB
C albumin and protein
D cytology
E glucose

72. A 45-year-old woman presents with severe itching, recent pale stools and dark urine. On examination there is darkened skin pigmentation, xanthelasma and hepatomegaly. Her test results are as follows

Serum bilirubin	15 μmol/L
Serum alkaline phosphatase	400 IU/L (30–300 IU/L)
AST	40 IU/L (5–35 IU/L)

The SINGLE best test to confirm the diagnosis is

A serum antimitochondrial antibody
B hepatitis virology
C liver biopsy
D Kveim test
E abdominal ultrasound

73. A 60-year-old man presents with increasing abdominal girth. On examination you elicit shifting dullness. The ascitic fluid tap reveals straw-coloured fluid containing 50 g/L of protein and elevated LDH. It contains 1000 WBC's/mm^3 (no lymphocytes) and many red cells are present. His serum total protein is 40 g/L. The MOST likely diagnosis is

A cirrhosis
B tuberculosis
C malignancy
D pancreatitis
E hepatic vein obstruction

74. A 55-year-old man complains of rectal bleeding. He is noted to have freckles on his lips. His father had undergone bowel surgery but he is not sure why. The MOST likely diagnosis is

A Crohn's disease
B ulcerative colitis
C Peutz–Jegher syndrome
D hereditary haemorrhagic telangiectasia
E familial adenomatous polyposis

75. A 40-year-old woman presents with a right-sided pleural effusion and ascites. Abdominal ultrasound reveals a left ovarian mass. The MOST likely diagnosis is

A pseudomyxoma peritonei
B Meig's syndrome
C Budd–Chiari syndrome
D nephrotic syndrome
E tuberculosis

76. A 44-year-old woman presents with fatigue and ascites. She is noted to have an irregular pulse of 120 with small volume. The chest x-ray is unremarkable. The 12-lead ECG demonstrates atrial fibrillation with low QRS voltage and T-wave inversion. The MOST likely diagnosis is

A right heart failure due to mitral stenosis
B Budd–Chiari syndrome
C constrictive pericarditis
D primary pulmonary hypertension
E tuberculous peritonitis

77. A 50-year-old woman presents with watery diarrhoea and right iliac fossa pain. On examination a rumbling mid-diastolic murmur is auscultated at the lower left sternal border, louder on inspiration, and the liver is enlarged. 12-lead ECG shows peak, tall P waves in lead II. The MOST useful investigation would be

A serum gastrin
B urine 5-hydroxy-indole acetic acid
C serum vasoactive intestinal peptide (VIP)
D urine vanillyl-mandelic acid
E fasting calcium

78. A 60-year-old man presents with persistent fever, profuse watery diarrhoea and crampy abdominal pain for the past week. He has just completed treatment for osteomyelitis. Proctosigmoidoscopy reveals erythematous ulcerations and yellowish-white plaques. The MOST likely diagnosis is

A ulcerative colitis
B Crohn's disease
C pseudomembranous colitis
D viral gastroenteritis
E Clostridium perfringens enterocolitis

79. A 40-year-old woman presents with abdominal bloating, diarrhoea and weight loss for 9 months. She had last felt really well on holiday in Tunisia over a year ago. Results show:

White cell count	11×10^9/L
Hb	9 gm/dL
Platelets	150×10^9/L
Blood film	microcytes and macrocytes, hypersegmented neutrophils
	Howell-Jolly bodies

The MOST likely diagnosis is

A Crohn's disease
B tropical sprue
C coeliac disease
D giardiasis
E Whipple's disease

80. A 66-year-old woman presents in a coma. Temperature 35°C, pulse 50 and BP 140/80. On examination she has a goitre and few basal rales in the chest. Her deep tendon reflexes are not brisk. Her medications are thyroxine, bendrofluazide, and omeprazole. Blood results:

Plasma sodium	129 mmol/L
Plasma potassium	3.6 mmol/L
Plasma urea	10 mmol/L
Plasma creatinine	130 μmol/L
Plasma glucose	3 mmol/L

The MOST appropriate medication would be

A propranolol
B frusemide
C triiodothyronine
D dextrose infusion
E hydrocortisone sodium succinate

81. A 16-year-old girl presents with an anterior neck mass. It moves on protrusion of her tongue. Thyroid radionucleotide scan shows no uptake in the midline. The MOST likely diagnosis is

A lingual thyroid
B Hashimoto's thyroiditis
C thyroglossal cyst
D thyroid follicular adenoma
E Riedel's thyroiditis

82. A 50-year-old woman who underwent a thyroidectomy a week ago now presents with confusion. She also complains of perioral tingling. The MOST discriminating investigation is

A serum glucose
B liver function tests
C full blood count and film
D thyroid function tests
E serum calcium

83. A 60-year-old man presents to Casualty drowsy and confused. Blood test results:

Serum sodium	150 mmol/L
Serum potassium	5 mmol/L
Serum chloride	105 mmol/L
Serum bicarbonate	30 mmol/L
Serum urea	10 mmol/L
Serum glucose	40 mmol/L

The following management is advisable EXCEPT

A 0.9% saline IVI
B heparin
C insulin at 3 U/h
D measure serum potassium hourly
E blood cultures

84. A 50-year-old man complains of loss of libido. He takes humulin and actrapid insulin. He is noted to have an enlarged liver. The MOST discriminating investigation is

A serum copper and caeruloplasmin
B serum gamma-glutamyl transferase
C HbsAg
D serum iron and total iron binding capacity
E mitochondrial antibodies

85. An 18-year-old female, who recently started the combined oral contraceptive pill on holiday in Kenya, complains of colicky abdominal pain, vomiting and fever. She develops progressive weakness in her extremities. The MOST likely diagnosis is

A acute pyelonephritis
B acute intermittent porphyria
C ureteric calculus
D malaria
E systemic lupus erythematosis

86. A 20-year-old female presents with acne and hirsutism. She complains of a year of chaotic menstrual cycles with long periods of amenorrhoea. She has gained weight recently. She has never been pregnant. On examination there are no other abnormalities. The MOST appropriate initial investigation would be

A laparoscopy
B 24-hour urinary free cortisol
C serum 17-hydroxyprogesterone levels
D serum LH, FSH and testosterone levels
E chromosome karyotyping

87. A 45-year-old obese man is noted to have glycosuria. He has no symptoms. Diabetes is confirmed on oral glucose tolerance test. The MOST appropriate management for this patient is

A commence biguanide
B commence sulphonylurea
C advise on diet and exercise
D commence on humulin and actrapid insulin
E admit to hospital

88. 60-year-old woman presents with a firm nodular midline neck mass. Blood tests reveal the presence of antibody to thyroglobulin and low serum thyroxine. The CORRECT diagnosis is

A Grave's disease
B deQuervain's thyroiditis
C Riedel's thyroiditis
D Hashimoto's thyroiditis
E thyroid carcinoma

89. A 70-year-old woman presents with recent onset of urinary incontinence. The MOST appropriate initial investigation is

A MSU for dipstick
B urodynamics
C full blood count
D serum urea and electrolytes
E MSU for culture and sensitivities

90. A 65-year-old diabetic man presents with a painless distended bladder. His urine dipstick shows no evidence of infection. The MOST useful investigation is

A excretion urography
B retrograde ureterography
C serum urea and electrolytes
D cystourethroscopy
E pressure-flow studies

91. A 40-year-old man presents with proteinuria, haematuria and progressive renal failure. He is also noted to have a high frequency sensorineural hearing loss. He has a sister who was noted to have microscopic haematuria but is asymptomatic now. The MOST likely diagnosis is

A membranous glomerulonephritis (GN)
B Alport's syndrome
C Goodpasture's syndrome
D Wegener's granulomatosis
E focal glomerulosclerosis

92. A 60-year-old man presents with fits and confusion. He has a past history of myocardial infarction and bowel resection. On chest examination there are bilateral rales and crackles. There has been no urine output from his Foley catheter. His serum urea is 50 mmol/L and his potassium is 8 mmol/L. The FIRST MOST appropriate step would be

A 15 units of soluble insulin with 50 g glucose (50%) IV
B 10–30 ml IV calcium gluconate (10%)
C continuous arteriovenous haemofiltration
D haemodialysis
E bicarbonate (100 mls of a 4.2% solution) by IVI

93. A 45-year-old well-controlled insulin-dependent diabetic is pre-scribed captopril for hypertension. He has a history of intermittent claudication and suffers rest pain. There is 3+ proteinuria. Urea and creatinine are elevated. On examination there is an abdominal bruit. The MOST likely diagnosis for his renal condition is

A diabetic nephropathy
B focal segmental glomerulosclerosis
C renal artery stenosis
D membranous glomerulonephritis
E renal cholesterol embolism

94. A 50-year-old woman presents with flaccid bullae over her trunk and limbs. She takes penicillamine and diclofenac for her rheumatoid arthritis. The MOST likely diagnosis for her skin condition is

A bullous pemphigoid
B pemphigus vulgaris
C epidermolysis bullosa
D dermatitis herpetiformis
E systemic lupus erythematosus

95. A 60-year-old woman presents with a slowly-growing, painless but itchy flat red scaly plaque on her lateral lower calf. The MOST use-ful investigation would be

A skin scrapings
B skin biopsy
C serum glucose
D none – spot diagnosis
E sentinel node biopsy

96. Stevens–Johnson syndrome is associated with all of the following drugs EXCEPT

    A penicillin
    B sulphonamides
    C oral contraceptives
    D thiazide diuretics
    E salicylates

97. A 65-year-old farmer presents with a grey thickened patch of skin on the rim of his left ear. The 1-cm lesion is painless, raised, firm, and has not changed in size over many years. The MOST likely diagnosis is

    A basal cell carcinoma
    B keratoacanthoma
    C solar keratosis
    D seborrhoeic keratosis
    E squamous cell carcinoma

98. A 20-year-old man presents with a brown discoloured toenail. On examination there is nail pitting and brown pigmentation at the base of the great toe-nail and the cuticle. He states that the colour started under the nail and has spread down to his nail-bed. The MOST likely diagnosis is

    A subungual haematoma
    B psoriasis
    C paronychia
    D melanoma
    E onychomycosis

99. A 30-year-old woman presents with a solitary painless genital ulcer with a hard, indurated base. The MOST useful investigation of the lesion is

    A Gram stain
    B dark field microscopy
    C virology
    D saline mount
    E biopsy

100. A 20-year-old man complains of urethral discharge and lesions on his palms and penis. He also complains of itchy burning eyes and pain in his right knee. On examination you note crusty scaling papules on his palms and glans penis. Subungual cornified material is seen but no nail pitting. The MOST likely diagnosis is

A gonorrhoea infection
B Reiter's syndrome
C Behçet's syndrome
D chlamydia infection
E psoriasis

Answers to Paper One BOFs

Criterion Referencing Marks

*   – 25–50% of candidates expected to get correct
**   – 50–75% of candidates expected to get correct
***   – 75–100% of candidates expected to get correct

The notional PASS MARK is 76%

1. C *** The rash is erysipelas.

2. B *** Trichomonas vaginalis is associated with a "strawberry" cervix. Wet film demonstrates the flagellated organism.

3. D ***

4. B * Rifampicin should be avoided in the presence of anti-retroviral drugs.

5. C ***

6. B ** The patient has malaria.

7. D **

8. D **

9. B ***

10. C *** The diagnosis of Hodgkin's disease is best made by lymph node biopsy. Bronchoscopy in the present of SVC obstruction to evaluate for bronchial carcinoma is ill-advised.

11. A ***

12. C ***

13. B **

14. B ** Seminomas are radiosensitive.

15. D **

16. B *** The patient has multiple myeloma.

17. C ***

18. B *

19. B ** Isoniazid is associated with B6 deficiency.

20. A ***

21. A ** Propranolol has a hypoglycaemic-effect and also masks the autonomic response to hypoglycaemia.

22. B ***

23. A *** Warfarin is used in rat poison.

24. A **

25. D **

26. D *

27. A **

28. E ***

29. E *

30. B * She has psoriatic arthropathy.

31. A ***

32. C *** On examination the disappearing murmur is known as the Carey-Coombs murmur.

33. E ***

34. C **

35. B ***

36. B ***

37. A ***

38. D ***

39. E **

40. E **

41. C ***

42. C ***

43. D *

44. B **

45. C ***

46. C **

47. A *** This is classic farmer's lung. Dairy farmers require hay to feed their cows.

48. D ***

49. B ** The common peroneal nerve may be injured at the neck of the fibula.

50. D *

51. E *** The patient has syphilis.

52. B *** The patient has a subdural haematoma.

53. E ***

54. D **

55. C ***

56. E *** The patient has vitamin B_{12} deficiency.

57. D *** Also known as lateral medullary syndrome.

58. C * This is a case of optic atrophy induced by tobacco due to cyanide poisoning and exacerbated by vitamin B_{12} deficiency.

59. C ***

60. C * This patient has limbal ischaemia and warrants urgent ophthamologist referral as the patient is at risk of corneal necrosis in <24 hours!

61. C ***

62. B *** MRI is likely to show patchy demyelination characteristic of multiple sclerosis.

63. C *** The patient has Kaposi's sarcoma.

64. A ***

65. B ***

66. B ***

67. B ***

68. D ***

69. B ***

70. C *** Grey–Turner's sign is associated with acute pancreatitis.

71. E ***

72. A ***

73. C **

74. C ***

75. B ***

76. C ***

77. B ***

78. C ***

79. C ***

80. C ***

81. C **

82. E ***

83. A *** 0.45% saline should be used if the Na is >150.

84. D **

85. B **

86. D **

87. C ***

88. D ***

89. A ***

90. E **

91. B **

92. B ***

93. C *** ACE inhibitors should be avoided in silent atherosclerosis, in particular, renal artery stenosis and may precipitate acute renal failure if administered.

94. B ** Pemphigus vulgaris is precipitated by penicillamine.

95. B ** The lesion is probably Bowen's disease.

96. C **

97. C ***

98. D **

99. B *** The patient has a syphilitic chancre.

100. B ***

Questions

1. Recognised causes of hypercalcaemia include

   A thiazide diuretics
   B hypoparathyroidism
   C milk alkali syndrome
   D hypothyroidism
   E vitamin D intoxication

2. X-linked diseases include

   A Christmas disease
   B achondroplasia
   C retinitis pigmentosa
   D Duchenne's muscular dystrophy
   E hypophosphataemic rickets

3. Immune complex mediated diseases include

   A SLE
   B primary biliary cirrhosis
   C diabetes mellitus
   D Goodpasture's syndrome
   E Rhesus incompatibility

4. The following hypersensitivity reactions and examples are correctly matched

   A Type I – ABO incompatibility
   B Type II – idiopathic thrombocytopaenic purpura
   C Type II – tuberculosis
   D Type III – Goodpasture's syndrome
   E Type IV – urticaria

5. Recognised causes of amyloidosis include

   A bronchiectasis
   B cirrhosis
   C multiple myeloma
   D osteomyelitis
   E rheumatoid arthritis

6. Amyloid is

   A a soluble protein
   B an intracellular protein
   C arranged in alpha-pleated configuration
   D associated with multiple myeloma
   E is diagnosed by Congo red staining of a rectal biopsy

7. Tumour necrosis factor (cachectin)

   A is triggered by interleukin-2
   B stimulates the release of leukotrienes and prostaglandins
   C is released from macrophage and lymphocyte-derived cytokines
   D is triggered by bacterial endotoxin (LPS)
   E is triggered by C5a

8. The following are protease inhibitors used for the treatment of HIV infection

   A indinavir
   B lamivudine
   C didanosine
   D efavirenz
   E ritonavir

9. Recognised features of glandular fever (infectious mononucleosis) include

   A Bell's palsy
   B leukopaenia
   C palatal petechiae
   D pericarditis
   E rash with administration of ampicillin

10. The following statements regarding typhoid fever are correct

    A may be complicated by osteomyelitis
    B has a mortality rate of 90% if left untreated
    C presents with abdominal pain and bloody diarrhoea
    D rose spots occur in the majority of patients
    E is caused by Salmonella typhi

11. Hepatitis A infection is associated with

    A an incubation period of up to 2 weeks
    B eating shellfish
    C presence of IgG antibody in recent infection
    D faecal-oral route of transmission
    E jaundice is present in most cases

12. Causes of megaloblastic erythropoiesis include

    A alcoholic liver disease
    B coeliac disease
    C hypothyroidism
    D sideroblastic anaemia
    E vegan diet

13. Non-metastatic effects of bronchial carcinoma include

    A acanthosis nigricans
    B hypertrophic pulmonary osteoarthropathy
    C myasthenic syndrome
    D nephrotic syndrome
    E leuconychia

14. Haemolytic anaemia is a recognised complication of the following drugs

    A co-trimoxazole
    B dapsone
    C diclofenac
    D penicillin
    E pyridoxine

15. The following tumour markers and tumours are correctly matched

    A alkaline phosphatase – prostate carcinoma
    B alpha-fetoprotein – hydatidiform mole
    C carcino-embryonic antigen – gastric carcinoma
    D CA-125 – ovarian carcinoma
    E human chorionic gonadotrophin – choriocarcinoma

16. Pernicious anaemia is associated with

    A increased incidence of pancreatic carcinoma
    B myxoedema
    C splenomegaly
    D mental confusion
    E jaundice

17. Potential side-effects of phenothiazine-derived antipsychotic drugs include

    A diarrhoea
    B haemolytic anaemia
    C hypertension
    D neuroleptic malignant syndrome
    E tardive dyskinesia

18. Drugs that induce hepatic enzyme activity significantly affecting their efficacy include

A carbamazepine
B doxycycline
C phenytoin
D rifampicin
E warfarin

19. Metronidazole is used in the treatment of

A actinomycosis israelii
B chlamydia trachomatis
C giardiasis
D Helicobacter pylori
E leptospirosis

20. The following pairs of drug poisoning and antidotes are matched correctly

A carbamazepine – N-acetylcysteine
B heparin – phytomenadione
C iron – dicobalt edetate
D paracetamol – activated charcoal
E diazepam (valium) – flumazenil

21. Gingival hypertrophy is a recognised side-effect of the following drugs

A cyclosporin
B lead poisoning
C methotrexate
D nifedipine
E phenytoin

22. Aortic regurgitation may be associated with

A ankylosing spondylitis
B ASD ostium primum
C infective endocarditis
D Marfan's syndrome
E thyrotoxicosis

23. Phaeochromocytoma

A are bilateral in 10% of cases
B often present with glycosuria
C occur in the adrenal cortex in the majority of cases
D may require phenoxybenzamine and propranolol to control BP
E may be autosomal dominantly inherited

24. In coronary artery bypass graft (CABG) surgery

    A graft patency rates with the left internal mammary artery are higher than with the saphenous vein
    B personality change is a recognised complication
    C CABG has equal efficacy as percutaneous transluminal coronary angioplasty (PTCA)
    D mortality rate is 5%
    E left main stem disease is a recognised indication

25. Hereditary angio-oedema

    A has an autosomal recessive inheritance
    B is associated with C1-esterase inhibitor deficiency
    C may present with abdominal pain
    D is treated with danazol
    E attacks may be preceded by erythema multiforme rash

26. Features of uncomplicated mitral stenosis include

    A middiastolic murmur at the apex
    B loud second heart sound
    C right ventricular hypertrophy
    D midsystolic murmur at the apex
    E haemoptysis

27. The following conditions are associated with conductive hearing loss

    A otosclerosis
    B Meniere's disease
    C acoustic neuroma
    D nasopharyngeal carcinoma
    E chronic secretory otitis media

28. Causes of wasting of the small muscles of the hand include

    A carpal tunnel syndrome
    B muscular dystrophy
    C myasthenia gravis
    D peripheral neuropathy
    E rheumatoid arthritis

29. Causes of monocular loss of vision include

    A carotid artery atheromatous plaque
    B disseminated sclerosis
    C epidural haematoma
    D subarachnoid haemorrhage
    E temporal arteritis

30. Features of temporal lobe disease may include

A aphasia
B auditory hallucinations
C automatism
D olfactory hallucinations
E lower homonymous quadrantanopsia

31. Recognised features of Wernicke's encephalopathy include

A altered consciousness
B ataxic gait
C external recti ophthalmoplegia
D horizontal nystagmus
E ptosis

32. Loss of consciousness may be associated with

A syndrome of inappropriate ADH
B lassa fever
C typhoid fever
D Guillain–Barré syndrome
E schistosomiasis

33. Neuropathic joints may be found in

A leprosy
B tabes dorsalis
C syringomyelia
D multiple sclerosis
E motor neurone disease

34. A pedestrian involved in a road traffic accident (RTA) fails to regain consciousness. Possible causes include

A fat embolism
B myocardial infarction
C extradural haematoma
D pulmonary embolism
E cardiac tamponade

35. CD4 lymphocytes

A recognise cells having major histocompatability Class II antigens
B secrete interleukin I in response to antigenic stimulation
C play a role in cellular immunity
D are associated with suppresser T cells
E have a receptor for HTLV-3

36. Features of portal hypertension include

    A splenomegaly
    B hypoalbuminaemia
    C ascites
    D encephalopathy
    E gastric varices

37. Steatorrhoea is a recognised feature of

    A ankylostomiasis
    B Crohn's disease
    C giardiasis
    D multiple jejunal diverticula
    E ulcerative colitis

38. Recognised associations of gluten-sensitive enteropathy (coeliac disease) include

    A aphthous mouth ulcers
    B carcinoma of the oesophagus
    C dermatitis herpetiformis
    D pyoderma gangrenosum
    E renal oxalate stones

39. Gastro oesophageal reflux disease (GORD) is associated with

    A anorexia nervosa
    B Helicobacter pylori
    C rolling hiatal hernia
    D systemic sclerosis
    E squamous carcinoma of the oesophagus

40. Acute cholecystitis may be associated with

    A absence of gallstones
    B back pain
    C hyperactive bowel sounds
    D pruritis
    E reflux oesophagitis

41. Recognised causes of portal hypertension include

    A inferior vena cava thrombosis
    B myelofibrosis
    C sarcoidosis
    D portal vein thrombosis
    E primary biliary cirrhosis

42. Primary biliary cirrhosis

   A is associated with dry eyes
   B is associated with raised serum IgA levels
   C is associated with night blindness
   D has raised liver copper in the early stages
   E is frequently associated with presence of endomysial antibodies

43. Vitamin B_{12} deficiency may result from

   A Crohn's disease
   B coeliac disease
   C highly selective vagotomy
   D jejunal diverticulosis
   E ulcerative colitis

44. Atrial natriuretic peptide (ANP)

   A increases renin secretion
   B decreases glomerular filtration rate
   C increases water and sodium excretion from the kidney
   D increases aldosterone secretion
   E is a powerful vasodilator

45. Prostacyclin

   A causes pulmonary vasoconstriction
   B activates platelets
   C is found in the endothelial and smooth muscle cells of vessel walls
   D is unaffected by aspirin
   E is formed from PGG2 (cyclic endoperoxide)

46. Paget's disease (osteitis deformans) is associated with

   A hypocalcaemia
   B normal bone turnover
   C severe bone pain alleviated by intravenous disodium pamidronate
   D pathological fractures
   E nerve deafness

47. Causes of keratoconjunctivitis sicca include

   A thyroiditis
   B primary biliary cirrhosis
   C myaesthenia gravis
   D Bell's palsy
   E pemphigus

48. In hyperthyroidism

    A Grave's disease accounts for 50% of cases
    B radioactive iodine has potential risks of hyperparathyroidism
    C severe cases may mimic acute abdomen
    D there is an increased incidence among males
    E treatment is with carbimazole 20 mg bd for up to one year

49. Recognised complications of diabetes mellitus include

    A loss of libido
    B orthostatic hypotension
    C nephrotic syndrome
    D nocturnal diarrhoea
    E reflux oesophagitis

50. Anovulatory cycles are associated with

    A climacteric
    B dysfunctional uterine bleeding
    C increased risk of cervical carcinoma
    D infertility
    E regular duration

51. Scant body hair is associated with

    A panhypopituitarism
    B anorexia nervosa
    C Cushing's syndrome
    D Turner's syndrome
    E Klinefelter's syndrome

52. Painless haematuria is a characteristic feature of

    A hydronephrosis
    B renal tuberculosis
    C transitional cell tumour of the bladder
    D cystitis
    E porphyria

53. Complications of thiazide diuretics include

    A hypocalcaemia
    B hypoglycaemia
    C hypouricaemia
    D intrahepatic cholestasis
    E metabolic acidosis

54. Features of rheumatoid arthritis include

    A Heberden's nodes
    B painful subcutaneous nodules
    C early morning stiffness
    D symmetrical synovitis
    E fibrosing alveolitis

55. Gout may be precipitated by

    A aspirin
    B eating roast goose
    C excess exercise
    D surgery under local anaesthesia
    E thiazide diuretics

56. Recognised features of SLE include

    A anti-neutrophil cytoplasmic antibody positive
    B hepatomegaly
    C normochromic normocytic anaemia
    D psychosis
    E rheumatoid factor negative

57. Recognised features of Marfan's syndrome include

    A aortic incompetence
    B autosomal dominant inheritance
    C lens dislocation
    D mental retardation
    E osteoporosis

58. Features of temporal arteritis (giant cell arteritis) include

    A bitemporal hemianopsia
    B dysarthria
    C scalp tenderness
    D seizure
    E temporomandibular joint instability

59. Features of polymyalgia rheumatica (PMR) may include

    A angina
    B depression
    C hyperparathyroidism
    D morning stiffness in the distal muscles
    E pulmonary infarcts

60. Tongue abnormalities are found in:

    A acromegaly
    B amyloidosis
    C CREST syndrome
    D motor neurone disease
    E vitamin B$_1$ deficiency

Answers to Paper Two MCQs

Criterion Referencing Marks

*   – 25–50% of candidates expected to get correct
**   – 50–75% of candidates expected to get correct
***   – 75–100% of candidates expected to get correct

The notional PASS MARK is 216/300 or 72%

---

1. TFTFT *** Causes of hypercalcaemia include hyperparathyroidism and thyrotoxicosis.

2. TFTTT **

3. TTTTF **

4. FTFFF * Goodpasture's syndrome and ABO incompatibility are examples of a Type II (cytotoxic) hypersensitivity reaction. Urticaria is an example of a type I reaction. Tuberculosis is an example of delayed hypersensitivity Type IV reaction.

5. TFTTT **

6. FFFTT ** Amyloid is an extracellular protein arranged in beta-pleated manner.

7. FTTTT * TNF is triggered by IL-1 and plays an important role in endotoxic shock.

8. TFFFT * Lamivudine and didanosine (ddI) are nucleoside analogues or nucleoside reverse transcriptase inhibitors (NRTIs). Efavirenz is a NNRTI.

9. TFTTT *** Infectious mononucleosis is associated with lymphocytosis and a positive Monospot test. Ampicillin should be avoided.

10. TFFFT *** Enteric fever has a mortality of 10% if left untreated. Shigella infection presents with abdominal pain and bloody diarrhoea. Rose spots occur in 40% of patients.

11. FTFTF *** Hepatitis A has an incubation period of up to 6 weeks. IgM antibody represents recent infection. A prodrome of anorexia, fever, and joint pains precedes jaundice. However, jaundice may be absent.

12. FTFFT ** Hypothyroidism and sideroblastic anaemia are macrocytic anaemias with a normoblastic bone marrow.

13. FTTTF *** Leuconychia is associated with cirrhosis. Acanthosis nigricans is associated with stomach carcinoma.

14. TTTTF ** Pyridoxine is a form of treatment for haemolytic anaemia. Cotrimoxazole contains sulfamethoxazole. Another drug associated with haemolytic anaemia is sulfadiazine.

15. FFFTF * HCG is associated with hydatidiform moles and α-fetoprotein is associated with choriocarcinoma. Acid phosphatase is linked to prostate carcinoma.

16. FTTTT ** Pernicious anaemia is associated with an increased incidence of gastric carcinoma.

17. FTFTT **

18. TFTTF ** Doxycycline interferes with bowel flora. On a practical note, the combined oral contraceptive pill is less effective in the presence of hepatic enzyme inducers and antibiotics. Antibiotics impair the bacterial flora responsible for recycling of ethinyl-oestradiol from the large bowel.

19. TFTTF ***

20. FFFFT ** Iron poisoning is treated with desferrioxamine. Carbamazepine poisoning is treated with activated charcoal. Vitamin K is used to treat warfarin overdose not heparin. Paracetamol poisoning is treated with N-acetylcysteine.

21. TFFTT **

22. TFTTF ***

23. TFFTT ** 30% of cases present with glycosuria. 90% of cases occur in the adrenal medulla not cortex.

24. TTFFT **

25. FTTTF * Hereditary angio-odema is an autosomal dominant condition. It is associated with an erythema marginatum rash. The activity of hereditary angio-odema shows menstrual exacerbations.

26. TFFFT *** Mitral stenosis is associated with a loud first heart sound.

27. TFFTT ***

28. TTFTT ***

29. TTTFT **

30. TTTTF ** Olfactory hallucinations may result from damage to the medial temporal lobe or uncus.

31. TTTFT ** Wernicke's encephalopathy results from thiamine deficiency and is associated with vertical nystagmus, ophthalmoplegia and ataxia.

32. TTTFF ***

33. TTTFF ***

34. TTTTT **

35. TFTFT ** CD4 lymphocytes secrete interleukin 2 and are associated with T-helper cells.

36. TFTTT ***

37. FTTTF ***

38. TTTFF ** Other features of coeliac disease include anaemia, growth retardation, HLA-DR3 association (90%), osteomalacia, GI lymphoma, and oesophageal and gastric carcinoma.

39. FFFTF *** GORD is also associated with 3rd trimester pregnancy, oesophageal stricture, bile reflux and may mimic angina or exacerbate asthma.

40. TTFFF *** Acute cholecystitis arises from an impacted stone in the cystic duct. Acalculous cholecystitis can also arise where no stone is found at the time of surgery. Referred pain may result in back or shoulder tip pain. Bowel sounds may become absent. Jaundice results if there are co-existent common bile duct stones.

41. FTTTT ***

42. TFTFF *** PBC presents most commonly in middle-aged women. It is associated with raised serum IgM levels. Cholestyramine may worsen osteomalacia. The antimitochondrial antibody is present in 95% of cases.

43. TFFTF *** In coeliac disease, malabsorption occurs but not sufficient to deplete body stores.

44. FFTFT * ANP is secreted from atrial granules and acts on the kidney to increase water and sodium excretion and GFR. It decreases renin and aldosterone secretion. ANP plays an important role in cardiovascular and fluid balance.

45. FFTFT ** Prostacylin inhibits platelet aggregation and causes pulmonary and coronary vasodilatation. Asprin inhibits cyclooxygenase.

46. FFTTT *** Bone turnover is increased.

47. TTTFF ** Pemphigoid and not pemphigus is associated with dry eyes.

48. FFTFT *** Grave's disease accounts for 75% of cases of hyperthyroidism. Radioactive iodine may result in hypoparathyroidism.

49. FTTTT ***

50. TTFTF ** Anovulatory cycles are associated with irregular bleeding and prolonged endometrial stimulation. This puts the woman at risk for endometrial hyperplasia and endometrial carcinoma.

51. TFFFF ***

52. FTTFF **

53. FFFTF *** Thiazide diuretics may result in metabolic alkalosis. Other side-effects include hypomagnesaemia, hypokalaemia, hyperglycaemia, hypercalcaemia, hyperuricaemia and altered plasma lipid concentration.

54. FFTTT ***

55. TFTFT *** Gout may also be precipitated by purine-rich oily fish, obesity and secondarily by leukaemia, renal failure and polycythaemia.

56. FFTTF *** SLE is associated with a positive ANA not ANCA (Wegener's granulomatosis) and with splenomegaly not hepatomegaly.

57. TTTFF ***

58. FTTFF *** Temporal arteritis is associated with monocular blindness and jaw claudication.

59. FTFFT ** Features of PMR may include hypopituitarism and morning stiffness of the proximal muscles.

60. TTFTF *** Vitamin B_{12} deficiency is associated with a sore red tongue in 25% of cases.

In these questions candidates must select one answer only

Questions

1. A 23-year-old female with Hodgkin's disease presents with small, white mucosal flecks in her mouth that can be wiped off. The MOST appropriate management for this patient would be

   A betamethasone valerate cream
   B acyclovir
   C penicillin
   D oral nystatin
   E biopsy before initiating any of the above

2. A 30-year-old man with HIV presents with sudden bilateral painless loss of vision. The MOST likely cause is

   A Kaposi's sarcoma
   B candidiasis
   C chlamydia trachomatis
   D CMV retinitis
   E gonococcal infection

3. The organism MOST frequently isolated from the ascitic fluid of patients with spontaneous bacterial peritonitis is

   A Klebsiella sp.
   B Escherichia coli
   C Streptococcus pneumoniae
   D Bacteroides fragilis
   E Pseudomonas aeruginosa

4. A 20-year-old HIV-positive man presents with fever and meningism. CSF shows

Pressure	250 mm H_2O
WBCs	200/mm^3
Predom. Cells	lymphocytes
Glucose	33% plasma level
Protein	5 g/L

You suspect cryptococcal meningitis. Diagnosis is BEST confirmed by

A India ink stain of CSF
B CSF cryptococcal antigen
C culture of CSF
D blood culture
E Gomori methenamine-silver staining of culture

5. A 20-year-old college student presents with headache, ear ache and dry cough. The chest x-ray shows left lower lobe consolidation. White cell count is normal. The MOST likely pathogen is

A Streptococcus pneumoniae
B Klebsiella sp.
C Mycoplasma
D Haemophilus influenza
E Legionella pneumophila

6. A 17-year-old girl presents with meningism and conjunctival petechiae. The CSF is turbid with an abundance of polymorphs and protein. Gram-negative cocci are isolated. The MOST likely organism is

A Neisseria meningitidis
B Neisseria gonorrhoea
C Group B Streptococcus
D Haemophilus influenza
E Streptococcus pneumoniae

7. A 22-year-old woman, back from Thailand a fortnight ago, is rushed to casualty in a comatose state. On examination she is jaundiced and unrousable. Her reflexes are exaggerated. Blood results show

White cell count	4.0×10^9/L
Hb	4 g/dL, PCV 12%
Blood film	asexual forms, parasite count 10% of rbc's
Creatinine	265 μmol/L
Bilirubin	40 μmol/L
Blood glucose	2 mmol/L
Arterial blood gas:	pH 7.2, HCO_3 12 mmol/L, lactate 6 mmol/L

The MOST likely diagnosis is

A yellow fever
B African trypanosomiasis
C plasmodium falciparum malaria
D plasmodium ovale malaria
E plasmodium vivax malaria

8. The MOST appropriate treatment for this patient is

A give quinine dihydrochloride 10–20 mg/kg loading dose then 10 mg/kg 8 hourly IV
B administer IV fluids and supportive therapy
C give mefloquine in a stat dose of 15 mg/kg then 10 mg/kg 8 hours later
D give chloroquine
E give suramin 200 mg IV test dose and then 20 mg/kg IV on 5–10 occasions at 5-day intervals and add malarsoprol on day 8

9. A 50-year-old man presents with a lump in the posterior triangle of the neck. It has been present for 8 months and is associated with a cheesy serous discharge. The MOST likely diagnosis is

A squamous cell carcinoma
B tuberculous adenitis
C deep lobe of parotid tumour
D infected branchial cyst
E sebaceous cyst

10. A 60-year-old African man presents with bone pain. His blood results are

White cell count	3×10^9/L
Hb	9 gm/dL with rouleaux formation
Platelets	70×10^9/L
ESR	120 mm/h
Plasma calcium	2.8 mmol/L
Alkaline phosphatase	100 IU/L (30–300 IU/L)
Creatinine	300 µmol/L
Urea	10 mmol/L

The MOST likely diagnosis is

A sickle cell disease
B multiple myeloma
C thrombotic thombocytopaenic purpura
D polyarteritis nodosa
E primary hyperparathyroidism

11. A 22-year-old male presents with fever, sweating particularly at night, pruritus and weight loss. On examination he has palpable painless cervical lymph nodes and no skin manifestations. The MOST appropriate investigation would be

A full blood count
B lymph node biopsy
C chest x-ray
D CT scan of neck and mediastinum
E Mantoux test

12. The MOST likely diagnosis is

A tuberculosis
B Non-Hodgkin's lymphoma
C Hodgkin's lymphoma
D acute lymphoblastic leukaemia
E chronic lymphocytic leukaemia

13. A 50-year-old renal transplant recipient on immunosuppressive therapy with cyclosporin, azathioprine and prednisolone is MOST at risk of developing

A squamous cell carcinoma of the skin
B basal cell carcinoma of the skin
C lymphoma
D liver failure
E leukaemia

14. A 17-year-old man with known sickle cell disease presents with severe lower back pain. He has a history of seizures. The FIRST step in management should be

A give oxygen at 4 L/min via a face mask
B start IV fluids
C give pethidine 150 mg IM every 2 hours until the pain settles
D give morphine 1–2 mg IV every 2–3 minutes until the pain settles
E lumbar spine and pelvic x-ray

15. A 40-year-old man with a prosthetic heart valve on warfarin anticoagulation presents with haematuria. His INR is 4. The MOST appropriate management after withholding warfarin would be

A give 0.5–2 mg of vitamin K by slow IV injection
B no further treatment and recheck INR in 1–2 days
C commence heparin
D give 1 litre of FFP
E give prothrombin complex concentrate (Factor 9A) and Factor VII

16. Primary anti-phospholipid syndrome is associated with all of the following EXCEPT

A recurrent spontaneous abortion
B recurrent arterial thromboses
C recurrent venous thromboses
D thrombocytosis
E positive IgG anti-cardiolipin antibodies

17. Mulitiple myeloma is normally associated with all of the following EXCEPT

A β2-microglobulinuria
B high CRP
C high ESR
D urinary Bence–Jones protein
E high paraprotein levels

18. The BEST drug treatment for refractory ventricular fibrillation is

A adrenaline
B amiodarone
C lignocaine
D adenosine
E esmolol

19. Which ONE of the following drugs may induce a psychosis similar to paranoid schizophrenia?

   A heroin
   B ecstasy (methylenedioxy methamfetamine)
   C amphetamine
   D cocaine
   E barbiturates

20. A 25-year-old man presents to Casualty with repeated fits. He smells of alcohol and has jaw trismus. The MOST appropriate management is

   A give 100 mg of IV thiamine
   B give 50 ml of 50% glucose IV
   C give 10 mg IV diazepam over 2 min.
   D insert a Guedel oropharyngeal airway and prepare for endotracheal intubation
   E insert a nasopharyngeal airway and administer oxygen

21. A 40-year-old man presents to Casualty within one hour of a paracetamol overdose. He smells of alcohol. His family confirms that he drinks heavily but is not on any medication. 16 tablets are missing from his paracetamol packs. The MOST appropriate management would be

   A take emergency blood levels for paracetamol level
   B give oral DL-methionine 2.5 g immediately followed by 50 mg of activated charcoal
   C administer 50 mg of activated charcoal
   D give IV N-acetylcysteine 150 mg/kg in 200 ml of 5% dextrose over 15 min.
   E no treatment is required

22. A 55-year-old alcoholic is brought to Casualty by the police. He is confused and aggressive. There are no external signs of head trauma. Blood pressure is 140/90, heart rate 110, and he is pale. He has palmar erythema, tremors and smells of alcohol. The MOST important initial investigation for this man is

   A blood alcohol level
   B head CT scan
   C gamma glutamyl transferase
   D blood glucose
   E clotting screen

23. His blood pressure drops to 100/60, and he begins to vomit. The MOST appropriate management would be

    A set up an IVI and give chlormethiazole infusion 0.8% (8 mg/ml), 40–80 ml over 10 minutes
    B give IM vitamin B complex
    C arrange urgent head CT scan and inform neurosurgeons
    D endotracheal intubation and gastric lavage
    E give 10 mg metoclopramide IV

24. Recognised side-effects of heparin include the following EXCEPT

    A thrombosis
    B thrombocytopaenia
    C alopecia
    D osteoporosis
    E hypokalaemia

25. The following statements regarding statin lipid lowering drugs are correct EXCEPT

    A They should be initiated in patients with a coronary heart disease (CHD) risk >3% and with cholesterol concentrations >5 mmol/L.
    B They are advised for patients with triglyceride levels >5 mmol/L.
    C The upper age limit for initiating statin therapy for primary prevention is 69.
    D Pravastatin is the drug of choice for primary CHD prevention.
    E They act by inhibiting HMG CoA reductase.

26. The following statements regarding flecainide are correct EXCEPT

    A It blocks the inward sodium current in cardiac tissue.
    B It reduces automaticity.
    C It is safe in patients with heart failure.
    D It is a class I anti-arrhythmic drug.
    E It is used to terminate symptomatic acute atrial fibrillation of <48 hours.

27. A 50-year-old man complains of hardness of hearing and dyspnoea. He is noted to have a nasal septal perforation and a blood pressure of 140/90. His urinalysis shows red cells, protein and casts. The chest-x-ray reveals opacities. The SINGLE investigation which is of greatest diagnostic value is

    A cytoplasmic anti-neutrophil cytoplasmic antibody (c-ANCA)
    B perinuclear (p-ANCA)
    C antinuclear antibody
    D antibasement membrane antibodies
    E Mantoux test

28. A 50-year-old woman presents with rheumatoid arthritis and weight loss. On examination she is noted to have splenomegaly and increased skin pigmentation. She has a positive rheumatoid factor. Her blood tests show neutropenia and normochromic normocytic anaemia. The MOST likely diagnosis is

    A Sjogren's syndrome
    B SLE
    C Still's disease
    D Felty's syndrome
    E Caplan's syndrome

29. A 40-year-old woman complains of intolerance to cold weather and cold running water. On examination you note she has a beaked nose, radial furrowing of the lips and facial telangiectasiae. On examination of her hands you notice sausage-like digits and tapered fingers. The MOST likely diagnosis is

    A SLE
    B Sjogren's syndrome
    C systemic sclerosis
    D rheumatoid arthritis
    E dermatomyositis

30. A 55-year-old man presents with an acutely painful swollen right knee. He recently was prescribed bendrofluazide for mild hypertension. The MOST useful investigation would be

    A full blood count and ESR
    B viral antibodies including parvovirus
    C anti-nuclear antibody and rheumatoid factor
    D aspirate of joint effusion for gram stain and culture
    E aspirate of joint effusion for polarised light microscopy

31. A 25-year-old man presents to Casualty with sudden onset of severe lower back pain that radiates down his right leg. On examination he is noted to have scoliosis of the spine, limited spinal flexion, restricted straight leg raise, limited hip movements and sensory loss over the dorsum of the right foot. The MOST likely diagnosis is

    A spondylolisthesis
    B ankylosing spondylitis
    C acute cord compression
    D lumbar canal stenosis
    E lumbar disc prolapse

32. A 20-year-old woman presents with persistent cyanotic reticular mottling of the skin on the dorsum of her foot. The rash is accentuated in the cold. Temperature is 37.5°C, blood pressure 160/100, and trace proteinuria. Blood tests: elevated WBC with eosinophilia, normocytic normochromic anaemia and elevated ESR. The MOST likely diagnosis is

A Raynaud's phenomenon
B SLE
C polyarteritis nodosa
D rheumatoid arthritis
E Wegener's granulomatosis

33. The following auto-antibodies and diseases are correctly paired EXCEPT

A anti-striated muscle antibody – Dressler's syndrome
B anti-acetylcholine receptor antibody – myasthenia gravis
C anti-glomerular basement membrane antibody – Goodpasture's syndrome
D anti-intrinsic factor antibodies – pernicious anaemia
E p-ANCA – microscopic polyarteritis

34. The following statements regarding complement are correct EXCEPT

A Patients with hereditary angioedema have low levels of C1qEl.
B In gram-negative sepsis, C3 is low and C4 is normal.
C C3 nephritis factor is associated with membrano-proliferative glomerulonephritis.
D SLE is associated with low C3 and normal C4.
E Hereditary angioedema is associated with normal C3 and low C4.

35. The MOST useful initial screening test for SLE is

A anti-dsDNA antibody
B anti-nuclear antibody
C anti-cardiolipin antibody
D C3 and C4 levels
E anti-extractable nuclear antigen (ENA) antibody

36. Rheumatoid arthritis may be associated with all of the following EXCEPT

A ulnar deviation
B carpal tunnel syndrome
C Dupuytren's contracture
D painful flexor tenosynovitis
E trigger finger

37. Cardinal signs of flexor tendon sheath infection include all of the following EXCEPT

    A inability to move the digit
    B tenderness over the flexor tendon sheath
    C swelling
    D slight flexion
    E pain on passive extension of the digit

38. The diagnosis of acute recent myocardial ischaemia within minutes to 6 hours of the event is BEST confirmed by

    A clinical history and examination
    B presence of Q waves on 12-lead electrocardiogram
    C presence of ST-segment elevation and T-wave inversion on 12-lead electrocardiogram
    D elevated CK-MB enzymes
    E elevated cardiac troponins I and T

39. A 60-year-old man presents with chest pain and sudden onset of atrial fibrillation with a heart rate of 160/min. The MOST appropriate management would be

    A oxygen, heparin and synchronised DC shock
    B oxygen, heparin, IV amiodarone
    C oxygen, heparin, warfarin
    D oxygen, beta-blockers
    E oxygen, digoxin IV

40. Mitral regurgitation is BEST evaluated by

    A M-mode echocardiogram
    B 2D echocardiogram
    C 12-lead electrocardiogram
    D doppler echocardiography
    E thallium-201 nuclear scan

41. A 65-year-old man presents with an acute myocardial infarction with a new left bundle branch block. He had a haemorrhagic stroke a year ago. He is given 100% oxygen, diamorphine, metoclopramide, GTN and aspirin. The NEXT MOST appropriate management is

    A IV glycoprotein IIb/ IIIa inhibitor
    B thrombolytic therapy with streptokinase
    C coronary artery bypass surgery
    D percutaneous transluminal coronary angioplasty
    E continuous infusion of heparin

42. A 50-year-old man presents with dyspnoea on exertion. On examination he is noted to have distended neck veins, hepatomegaly and ascites. He is also noted to have a paradoxical pulse and a rising JVP on inspiration. Chest x-ray reveals a small heart with calcification. The MOST likely diagnosis is

   A viral pericarditis
   B tuberculous pericarditis
   C cardiac tamponade
   D malignant pericarditis
   E Dressler's syndrome

43. A 20-year-old woman presents with a BP of 170/100. On examination she has impalpable peripheral pulses, although systolic murmurs are auscultated above and below her clavicles. She also complains of diminishing vision and syncopal episodes. Her ESR is 50 mm/hr. The MOST likely diagnosis is

   A thrombangitis obliterans
   B coarctation of the aorta
   C Kawasaki's disease
   D Takayasu's disease
   E Raynaud's disease

44. A 35-year-old IV drug abuser presents with right upper quadrant abdominal pain. On examination he has peripheral oedema, ascites and a tender liver. On chest auscultation he has a pansystolic murmur along the left sternal border. The MOST likely diagnosis is

   A tricuspid regurgitation
   B ventricular septal defect
   C pulmonary stenosis
   D mitral regurgitation
   E tricuspid stenosis

45. A 60-year-old man in the Coronary Care Unit (CCU) has an elevated CVP reading a day after sustaining a myocardial infarction which is confirmed on two further quarter hourly readings. On examination he has a few basal creps. He is asymptomatic. The MOST appropriate management would be

   A give GTN, frusemide and an ACE inhibitor
   B advise no added salt in diet
   C give IV dopamine
   D insert a Swan-Ganz catheter to assess LV filling pressures
   E give 40 mg frusemide od

46. A 22-year-old woman presents with high blood pressure on routine physical examination. On examination she has a late systolic murmur and cold lower extremities. Her 12-lead ECG shows left ventricular hypertrophy. The MOST likely diagnosis is

    A coarctation of the aorta
    B systemic sclerosis
    C Takayasu's arteritis
    D Raynaud's disease
    E SLE

47. The BEST investigation to diagnose a pulmonary embolism is

    A arterial blood gases
    B ventilation-perfusion isotope scintigraphy
    C pulmonary angiogram
    D 12-lead electrocardiogram
    E PA and lateral chest x-ray

48. Which ONE of the following drugs is absolutely contraindicated in patients with asthma?

    A adenosine
    B atenolol
    C adrenaline
    D verapamil
    E bendrofluazide

49. A 60-year-old man has squamous cell carcinoma of the bronchus. The MOST useful investigation to assess curative surgical resection is

    A radionucleotide scanning for the detection of metastatic disease
    B fibreoptic bronchoscopy and cytology
    C CT scan of the mediastinum
    D measurement of FEV$_1$
    E transthoracic fine-needle aspiration biopsy of mediastinal lymph node

50. A 20-year-old man presents with recurrent sinusitis and recurrent otitis media. On CT scan of the sinuses, the frontal sinuses are maldeveloped. On chest x-ray there are cystic shadows with fluid levels and dextrocardia. His 12-lead ECG shows inverted P-waves in lead I and reversed R wave progression. The MOST likely diagnosis is

    A Down's syndrome
    B Kartagener's syndrome
    C Marfan's syndrome
    D cystic fibrosis
    E situs inversus

51. A 60-year-old man, with a history of COPD, presents to Casualty with a severe chest infection. On examination his temperature is 40°C, respiratory rate 32/minute, BP 120/55 and pulse rate is 110. Chest x-ray reveals a lobar pneumonia. He is not penicillin-allergic. The MOST appropriate therapy would be

A amoxycillin 500 mg o tds
B co-amoxyclavulanic acid 375 mg o tds + erythromycin 500 mg o qds
C cefotaxime 1–2 g IV tds + erythromycin 1g IV qds
D flucloxacillin 1–2 g IV qds + metronidazole 500 mg IV tds
E cefotaxime 1–2 g IV tds + gentamicin 2-5 mg/kg daily in 3 divided doses

52. Surgery for lung carcinoma is contraindicated in the presence of which ONE of the following?

A superior vena cava obstruction
B FEV$_1$ 2 L
C tumour involving the first 1 cm of either main bronchus
D hypertrophic pulmonary osteoarthropathy
E haemoptysis

53. A 50-year-old man with lymphadenopathy confined to the mediastinum and pleural effusion is diagnosed as tuberculosis. He is HIV positive. The BEST management option would be

A 2 months of rifampicin, isoniazid, pyrazinamide and ethambutol then 4 months of rifampicin and isoniazid
B full regimen for 2 months then 10 months of rifampicin and isoniazid
C standard above TB therapy plus corticosteroids
D omit rifampicin and extend TB treatment to 18 months
E standard above TB therapy but reduce the dose of ethambutol

54. A 20-year-old woman is found unconscious. The results of her blood tests are as follows

pH   7.2
Plasma sodium   139 mmol/L
Plasma potassium   4.2 mmol/L
Plasma chloride   102 mmol/L
Plasma HCO$_3$ 11 mmol/L

These results are MOST compatible with

A aspirin poisoning
B meningitis
C Addison's disease
D hyperosmolar non-ketotic coma
E subarachnoid haemorrhage

55. A 45-year-old man presents with ptosis, meoisis, and an unsteady gait. He is also noted to have bilateral gynaecomastia. The MOST likely diagnosis is

A alcoholism
B Klinefelter's syndrome
C heroin overdose
D Kallman's syndrome
E carcinoma of the lung

56. A 25-year-old man presents with weakness and numbness in his lower legs. He has just recovered from a recent chest infection. On examination deep tendon reflexes are absent and sensation is also lost. CSF from a lumbar puncture shows a normal cell count and glucose but raised protein level. The MOST likely diagnosis is

A mumps
B sarcoidosis
C AIDS
D Guillain–Barré syndrome
E Refsum's disease

57. The MOST useful step in guiding management would be

A pulse oximetry
B chest x-ray
C nerve conduction studies
D serial vital capacity
E serial peak flow measurement

58. A 50-year-old man presents with a sudden severe periorbital headache, neck pain and vomiting following sexual intercourse. The MOST useful investigation would be

A cerebral angiography
B carotid ultrasound and doppler examination
C head CT scan
D full blood count and urea and electrolytes
E lumbar puncture

59. A 30-year-old man presents with a unilateral facial nerve palsy that involves his forehead. Possible causes include the following EXCEPT

A Bell's palsy
B Ramsay–Hunt syndrome
C acoustic neuroma
D cerebrovascular accident
E parotid tumour

60. Carpal tunnel syndrome is associated with all of the following EXCEPT

A degenerative arthritis
B pregnancy
C acromegaly
D Colles' fracture
E Diabetes

61. Claw hand deformity may be seen with all of the following EXCEPT

A spinal cord injury
B Charcot–Marie–Tooth disease
C brachial plexus injuries
D combined median and ulnar nerve lesion
E rheumatoid arthritis

62. A 70-year-old man complains of flashing lights and floaters in his left eye for the past month and now complains of painless loss of vision in his left eye. The MOST likely diagnosis is

A central retinal artery occlusion
B central retinal vein occlusion
C optic neuritis
D retinal detachment
E macular degeneration

63. A 30-year-old man presents with a right red painful eye. He complains of watering of the eyes and sensitivity to light. He has a history of recurrent cold sores. The MOST appropriate treatment is

A prednisolone 0.5% 6 hourly
B acyclovir 3% eye ointment 5 times daily
C chloramphenicol 1% eye ointment
D acyclovir 800 mg 5 times daily
E cefuroxime 50 mg/ml

64. A 50-year-old woman presents with fever, headache, left eye pain and blurry vision. She states that she has just recovered from a cold. On examination she has a swollen left eyelid, mild proptosis and diminished visual acuity. She is unable to move her eye. The MOST likely diagnosis is

A orbital cellulitis
B giant-cell arteritis
C sinusitis
D choroiditis
E cavernous sinus thrombosis

65. A 20-year-old man presents with a painful red eye. He has a long history of backache. On examination you note pus in the anterior chamber and synechiae. The MOST likely diagnosis is

A ankylosing spondylitis
B Reiter's syndrome
C Crohn's disease
D sarcoidosis
E rheumatoid arthritis

66. The following are possible responses to grief EXCEPT

A anger
B denial
C catatony
D guilt
E delirium

67. A 60-year-old woman presents with progressive forgetfulness and mood changes. She has a shuffling gait. Her brain CT scan shows cortical atrophy and enlarged ventricles. Histology shows senile plaques and neurofibrillary tangles. The MOST likely diagnosis is

A Wernicke–Korsakoff syndrome
B Parkinson's disease
C Alzheimer's disease
D Variant Creutzfeldt–Jakob disease
E multi-infarct dementia

68. The following statements regarding venlafaxine are correct EXCEPT

A It has no affinity for adrenergic, cholinergic or histaminic receptors.
B It inhibits the reuptake of both serotonin and noradrenaline.
C MAOI's may be taken in conjunction with venlafaxine.
D It is effective against chronic and refractory depression.
E Nausea is the MOST common side-effect.

69. The following statements regarding anorexia nervosa are true EXCEPT

A A BMI of <13 warrants hospital admission.
B Anorexia is defined as a BMI <17.5 associated with food avoidance.
C Physical features include bradycardia and hypotension.
D Investigations are important in confirming the diagnosis.
E Anorexia may be associated with reduced bone mass.

70. A 40-year-old man presents with dysphagia and epigastric pain relieved by food and antacids. He has been taking NSAIDS for osteoarthritis of the hip for many months. On examination he has a palpable epigastric mass, a palpable supraclavicular lymph node. The MOST likely diagnosis is

A oesophageal squamous cell carcinoma
B duodenal ulcer
C peptic stricture of oesophagogastric junction
D gastric adenocarcinoma
E gastric ulcer

71. A 62-year-old man is admitted at 2AM with acute severe upper GI bleeding. On examination he is noted to have gynaecomastia and palmar erythema. His SBP is 90 and pulse 110. After starting him on IV gelofusin, ordering 6 units of blood and informing the duty surgeon, the NEXT MOST appropriate management would be

A emergency diagnostic endoscopy
B sedate wth I.V. diazepam
C give stat dose of 50 mcg IV octreotide followed by infusion at 50 mcg/hour
D insert gastroesophageal balloon to tamponade bleeding
E arrange OGD for the next routine list at 10 AM

72. A 25-year-old woman presents with 7 days of increasing bloody diarrhoea. She has just returned from Spain. On examination she has a temperature of 39°C and looks unwell. She is tender in the left lower quadrant of the abdomen. On proctoscopy it is difficult to see the mucosa, as it is obscured by blood and pus. The MOST appropriate management is

A send stool for microscopy and culture
B prescribe nightly hydrocortisone enema and oral mesalazine
C admit to hospital and ask GI surgeon to review
D prescribe tapering doses of oral prednisolone followed by olsalazine
E admit to hospital and arrange for urgent sigmoidoscopy and biopsies

73. A 50-year-old obese man presents complaining of recurrent abdominal pain radiating to the back and made worse by eating and bending over. Antacids relieve the pain. He smokes 20 cigarettes a day and drinks spirits daily. The MOST useful investigation would be

A oesophagogastroduodenoscopy
B double contrast barium meal
C Helicobacter pylori breath test
D abdominal ultrasound scan
E abdominal CT scan

74. The MOST likely diagnosis is

    A duodenal ulcer
    B gastro-oesophageal reflux disease (GORD)
    C acute pancreatitis
    D achalasia
    E Barrett's ulcer of the oesophagus

75. A 30-year-old man presents with crampy abdominal pain, diarrhoea and weight loss. On examination: temperature 39°C; no lymphadenopathy. Barium meal reveals a stricture in the terminal ileum. The MOST likely diagnosis is

    A tuberculosis
    B Crohn's disease
    C ulcerative colitis
    D lymphoma
    E coeliac disease

76. The BEST diagnostic test for Down's syndrome in a 10 week pregnant woman is

    A triple blood test for serum oestriol, α-fetoprotein, and β-human chorionic gonadotrophin
    B nuchal fold thickness scan
    C chorionic villus sampling
    D amniocentesis
    E chromosomal karyotyping of the parents

77. A 50-year-old man presents to Casualty with repeated fits. His plasma sodium is 112 mmol/L and urine osmolality is 550 mmol/kg. He is well hydrated. He smokes 20 cigarettes a day and drinks spirits daily. The MOST likely diagnosis is

    A SIADH
    B Addison's disease
    C liver cirrhosis
    D renal failure
    E diabetes insipidus

78. The MOST appropriate treatment to correct his hyponatraemia is

    A desmopressin
    B terlipressin
    C demeclocycline
    D hydrocortisone
    E chlorthalidone

79. A 40-year-old obese man with non-insulin dependent diabetes takes metformin bd. His HbA1C returns as 13%. The MOST appropriate management would be

A commence insulin therapy
B increase metformin to tds and add repaglinide
C switch to gliclazide 40 mg daily
D continue current dose of metformin
E repeat HbAIC in a month's time and advise diet and exercise

80. A 60-year-old man presents to casualty drowsy and confused. Blood test results

Serum sodium   150 mmol/L
Serum potassium   5 mmol/L
Serum chloride   105 mmol/L
Serum bicarbonate   30 mmol/L
Serum urea   10 mmol/L
Serum glucose   40 mmol/L

His serum osmolality IS

A 260 mmol/L
B 280 mmol/L
C 300 mmol/L
D 340 mmol/L
E 360 mmol/L

81. A 40-year-old woman presents with a painful neck swelling. She had a chest infection a week prior. On examination: temperature is 39°C. The thyroid gland is diffusely enlarged and tender. T3 and T4 are both elevated but the radio-iodine uptake is decreased. The MOST likely diagnosis is

A Riedel's thyroiditis
B Grave's disease
C follicular thyroid carcinoma
D DeQuervain's thyroiditis
E Hashimoto's thyroiditis

82. On general examination a 48-year-old man referred to the Diabetic Clinic has coarse oily skin and a prominent supraorbital ridge. He has widely-spaced teeth and a moist handshake. The man's general appearance is MOST likely to be due to

A acromegaly
B haemochromatosis
C Klinefelter's syndrome
D gigantism
E thyrotoxicosis

Paper Two BOF's questions

89

83. The following statements regarding oral hypoglycaemic agents are true EXCEPT

A Chlopropamide is associated with facial flushing after alcohol ingestion.
B Gliblencamide is associated with risk of serious hypoglycaemia in patients >70.
C Repaglinide acts by inhibition of ATP-dependent potassium ion channels.
D Metformin is the drug of first choice in obese patients in whom strict dieting has failed.
E Tolbutamide is a biguanide.

84. A 30-year-old female presents with severe headache and vomiting. She is sensitive to light and also complains of neck pain. BP is 170/110 and pulse 50. On examination she has bilateral ptosis, dilated pupils and eyes are positioned down and out. On fundoscopy bilateral papilloedema is present. Protein and glucose are present in her urine.

The most appropriate investigation is

A lumbar puncture
B head CT scan
C MRI scan of the brain
D cerebral angiography
E electroencephalogram

85. In normal pregnancy which ONE of the following is true?

A The average weight gain is 20 kg.
B Haemoglobin levels rise.
C A progressive rise in plasma creatinine occurs.
D The cardiac output rises to term.
E The glomerular filtration rate and renal plasma flow rise by ALMOST 50% by term.

86. Corticosteroid therapy reduces the progression towards renal failure in which ONE of the following conditions?

A post-streptococcal glomerulonephritis
B Berger's disease
C focal segmental glomerulosclerosis
D membranous glomerulonephritis
E rapidly progressive glomerulonephritis

87. You are called to see a 65-year-old woman with poor urine output. She is on IV flucloxacillin, benzylpenicillin and metronidazole for pelvic cellulitis. A Foley bladder catheter is inserted and the hourly urine output is confirmed as 10 ml/ hour. Her temperature is 38°C, blood pressure is 160/90 and pulse rate is 110. ECG shows peaked T waves and wide QRS complexes. Blood results include

Plasma sodium	139 mmol/L
Plasma potassium	6.9 mmol/L
Plasma urea	12 mmol/L
Plasma creatinine	300 μmol/L

The MOST appropriate management for this patient is

A administer a bolus of 1 litre of Hartmann's solution
B administer 20 ml of 10% calcium gluconate slowly into a central vein and administer 50 ml of 50% dextrose with 10 units of soluble human insulin over 30 min and thereafter at 10 ml/hr
C administer 50–100 ml of 8.45% $NaHCO_3$ slowly IV into a central vein
D administer 120 mg frusemide as a bolus dose IV
E take blood cultures

88. The urine osmolality is 550 mosm/L, and urine sodium is 15 mmol/L. The MOST likely cause for her acute renal failure is

A acute tubular necrosis
B hypovolaemia
C sepsis
D acute interstitial nephritis
E rapidly progressive glomerulonephritis

89. A 30-year-old woman presents with fever, cough and haematuria. She had been in Egypt 2 weeks previously. On examination she has hepatomegaly. The drug treatment of CHOICE is

A hycanthone
B praziquantel
C quinine
D rifampicin, isoniazid, pyrazinamide and ethambutol
E sodium stibocaptate

90. A 50-year-old man presents with a red scaly rash over his neck and trunk, which has not responded to a 1-month course of topical corticosteroids. On examination he has randomly distributed serpiginous annular red plaques over his trunk and cervical lymphadenopathy. Blood test results are

White cell count	20×10^9/L with 50% eosinophils
Hb	10 gm/dL
Platelets	150×10^9/L

The MOST likely diagnosis is

A psoriasis
B mycosis fungoides
C solar keratosis
D pityriasis rosea
E lichen simplex

91. A 25-year-old man presents with nonpruritic white spots on his trunk. On examination there are multiple sharply demarcated round depigmented macules of up to 2 cm in size. On gentle scratching, a delicate scaling is noted. There is no associated lymphadenopathy. There is no family history of depigmentation. The MOST useful investigation is

A potassium hydroxide preparation of skin scrapings and direct microscopic examination
B skin smears for AFB
C syphilis serology
D full blood count and film
E HLA-B markers

92. A 50-year-old diabetic man presents with a necrolytic migratory erythematous rash. The MOST likely explanation for the rash is

A somatostatinoma
B vipoma
C glucagonoma
D insulinoma
E gastrinoma

93. A 60-year-old woman presents with a slowly-growing, painless but itchy flat red scaly plaque on her lateral lower calf. The MOST likely diagnosis is

A psoriasis
B granuloma annulare
C Bowen's disease
D squamous cell carcinoma
E necrobiosis lipoidica

94. A 50-year-old woman who is an avid sunbather presents with a red forehead with scaly rash. On examination, the lesions are multiple, discrete, small, erythematous, with a keratotic surface and varying from a few millimetres to up to 1 cm in diameter. The lesions are gritty to the touch. The MOST likely diagnosis is

A squamous cell carcinoma
B actinic keratosis
C discoid lupus erythematosus
D seborrheic keratosis
E psoriasis

95. A 50-year-old woman who is an avid sunbather presents with a red forehead with scaly rash. On examination, the lesions are multiple, discrete, small, erythematous, with a keratotic surface and varying from a few millimetres to up to 1 cm in diameter. The lesions are gritty to the touch. The woman has tried topical diclofenac with no improvement. The next MOST appropriate treatment for this woman is

A curettage
B topical fluorouracil (efudix)
C cryotherapy
D tangential excision
E photodynamic therapy

96. A 40-year-old man presents with a new intertriginous rash in both axillae. The area shows brown pigmentation in areas of multiple confluent papillomas. The rash is sometimes itchy. The MOST likely diagnosis for his rash is

A acanthosis nigricans
B dermatomyositis
C Addisonian hyperpigmentation
D porphyria cutanea tarda
E malignant melanoma

97. In the management of HIV in pregnancy, which ONE of the following drugs is CONTRAINDICATED?

A efavirenz
B lamivudine
C ritonavir
D zidovudine
E nelfinavir

98. Prophylaxis against opportunistic infections is advised when the CD4 count falls BELOW

A 500 cells/mm^3
B 300 cells/mm^3
C 250 cells/mm^3
D 200 cells/mm^3
E 100 cells/mm^3

99. All the following are opportunistic infections in HIV disease EXCEPT

A mycobacterium avium
B toxoplasma gondii
C pneumocystis carinii
D cytomegalovirus
E Helicobacter pylori

100. 20-year-old homosexual man presents with a greyish appearance at the lateral margins of the tongue. He does not drink or smoke and is not on any medication. The MOST likely infective cause is

A Epstein–Barr virus
B Candida albicans
C Treponema pallidum
D Herpes simplex
E HIV

Answers to Paper Two BOFs

Criterion Referencing Marks
*   – 25–50% of candidates expected to get correct
**   – 50–75% of candidates expected to get correct
*** ·– 75–100% of candidates expected to get correct

The notional PASS MARK is 77%

---

1. D ***

2. D ***

3. B ***

4. A ***

5. C ***

6. A ***

7. C **

8. A **

9. B ***

10. B ***

11. B *** The patient has Hodgkin's disease.

12. C ***

13. A **

14. D *** Seizures may be associated with pethidine.

15. C ** Vitamin K may induce prolonged warfarin resistance in patients with prosthetic heart valves.

16. D ** Primary anti-phospholipid syndrome is associated with thrombocytopaenia.

17. B *** Multiple myeloma is normally associated with low CRP. High CRP indicates concomitant infection.

18. B ***

19. C ***

20. E **

21. C **

22. D ***

23. A ***

24. E ** Heparin may be associated with hyperkalaemia and not hypokalaemia.

25. B **

26. C ** Flecainide is contraindicated in the presence of heart failure.

27. A *** 90% will have an increase in cANCA and 20–40% will have elevated p-ANCA.

28. D ***

29. C **

30. E ** This is a case of gout precipitated by thiazide diuretics.

31. E ***

32. C ** Livedo reticularis may be associated with PAN.

33. A *** Dressler's syndrome is associated with anti-cardiac muscle antibody.

34. D ** SLE is associated with low C3 and C4 levels.

35. B ***

36. C ***

37. A**

38. B ***

39. A **

40. D ***

41. D **

42. B ***

43. D ***

44. A *** The patient has infective endocarditis.

45. B ***

46. A ***

47. C ***

48. B ***

49. C **

50. B **

51. C ** The patient has a severe community-acquired pneumonia.

52. B ***

53. D *

54. A ***

55. E ***

56. D ***

57. D ***

58. C *** Subarachnoid haemorrhage may present following sexual intercourse.

59. D ***

60. A ***

61. E **

62. D **

63. B **

64. A **

65. A ***

66. E ***

67. C ***

68. C * There should be a 14 day break between stopping MAOI's and commencing venlafaxine to avoid the serotonin syndrome.

69. D ***

70. D ***

71. A ***

72. E ***

73. A ***

74. B ***

75. B ***

76. C **

77. A ***

78. C ***

79. B **

80. E *** The formula for calculating the serum osmolality = 2 (Na + K) + glucose + urea

81. D **

82. A ***

83. E *** Tolbutamide is a sulfonylurea and metformin is a biguanide.

84. B ***

85. E **

86. D **

87. B ** The patient has prerenal failure.

88. C **

89. B ** Praziquantel available on named-patient basis.

90. B ***

91. A * The diagnosis is pityriasis versicolor alba.

92. C **

93. C ***

94. B ***

95. B *

96. A ***

97. A *

98. D **

99. E ***

100. A ***

MRCP Paper Three MCQs

Questions

1. The facial nerve
   A supplies taste sensation to the anterior 2/3 of the tongue
   B may be associated with hyperacusis if damaged
   C may cause loss of lacrimation due to involvement of the lesser petrosal nerve
   D if affected in upper motor neurone lesions results in paralysis of the forehead muscle
   E has three branches in the temporal bone

2. Recognised consequences of a median nerve lesion at the wrist include
   A wasting of the radial half of the hand
   B paralysis of opponens pollicis
   C loss of light touch over the radial three and a half fingers
   D wasting of the hypothenar eminence
   E wrist drop

3. Helicobacter pylori
   A is a Gram-positive organism
   B produces urease
   C is usually symptomatic at time of infection
   D is isolated in more patients with gastric rather than duodenal ulcers
   E has a predilection for the gastric antrum

4. Metabolic alkalosis is associated with
   A early stages of aspirin poisoning
   B chronic renal failure
   C milk alkali syndrome
   D primary hyperaldosteronism
   E pyloric stenosis

5. The following congenital abnormalities are associated with a chromosomal abnormality

A Turner's syndrome
B Waardenburg's syndrome
C Edward's syndrome
D Patau's syndrome
E Treacher–Collins syndrome

6. The following statements are correct

A A double-blind study is when both doctor and patient are unaware of which treatment the patient is having.
B The prevalence of a disease is the number of cases, at any time during the study period, divided by the population at risk.
C Case-control studies are prospective.
D Case-control studies generate incidence data.
E A single-blind study is when the patient is not aware of which of the two treatments the patient is having.

7. The following statistical definitions are true

A The mean is the middle score of an ordered frequency distribution.
B The median is the value that occurs most often in a distribution.
C Negatively skewed distribution is one in which the mean is greater than the median.
D The variance is the average of the sum of square deviations.
E Standard deviation indicates what interval, measured from the mean, includes 34% of all observations in a normal distribution.

8. Hepatitis C virus

A is characterised by a mild acute infection
B is transmitted via blood transfusions
C infection is preventable with passive immunisation
D is transmitted via shared intravenous drug needles
E is less often associated with chronic hepatitis than hepatitis B

9. Antibiotic prophylaxis is required for a patient with a prosthetic mitral valve in the following instances

A IUCD insertion
B GI endoscopy
C barium enema
D cystoscopy
E dental scaling

10. Recognised complications of Mycoplasma pneumoniae infection include

A erythema marginatum
B myelitis
C diarrhoea
D myalgia
E Coombs' test negative haemolytic anaemia

11. Falciparum malaria in endemic areas

A should be treated with intravenous quinine if unable to be taken orally
B should be treated with Maloprim (pyremethamine and dapsone) as prophylaxis during early pregnancy
C can be prevented by chloroquine prophylaxis in coastal East Africa
D may be treated with oral quinine for 7 days followed by a stat dose of Fansidar (pyrimethamine and sulfadoxine)
E is the most common cause of benign malaria

12. Premalignant conditions include

A oral leucoplakia
B polycystic kidney disease
C xeroderma pigmentosa
D adenomatous polyposis coli
E bullous pemphigoid

13. Good prognostic factors for Hodgkin's lymphoma include

A male gender
B lymphocyte predominant histology
C involvement limited to single lymph node in the neck
D nodular sclerosing histology
E weight gain

14. Recognised features of aspirin poisoning include

A sensorineural hearing loss
B jaundice
C hypoventilation
D acute pancreatitis
E pupil constriction

15. Adverse side-effects of the combined oral contraceptive pill include

    A increased risk of thrombosis in blood group O
    B chorea
    C premenstrual tension
    D weight gain
    E irritation from contact lens

16. The following immunodeficiency diseases involve defective T-lymphocyte functions

    A hereditary angioedema
    B Job's syndrome
    C chronic granulomatous disease
    D Chediak–Higashi syndrome
    E Wiskott–Aldrich syndrome

17. Adrenaline

    A is the first drug used in cardiac arrest of any aetiology
    B is the second line treatment for cardiogenic shock
    C has solely alpha–adrenergic activity
    D cannot be administered via a tracheal tube
    E may be given as an alternative to external pacing in bradycardia

18. Concomitant use of the following pairs of drugs is contraindicated

    A verapamil and propranolol
    B gliclazide and warfarin
    C metronidazole and phenytoin
    D metoclopramide and paracetamol
    E thiazides and lithium

19. Amiodarone

    A decreases the duration of the action potential of both the atrial and ventricular myocardium
    B may be associated with hypothyroidism
    C is used to treat refractory ventricular fibrillation
    D may be associated with peripheral neuropathy
    E commonly causes reversible corneal microdeposits

20. Verapamil

    A increases conduction through the AV node
    B has a positive inotropic effect
    C may precipitate digoxin toxicity
    D may cause asystole in combination with beta-blockers
    E combined with a beta-blocker enhances the treatment of hypertension

21. Causes of acute pericarditis include

    A amyloidosis
    B coxsackie infection
    C myocardial infarction
    D thyrotoxicosis
    E uraemia

22. Large "a" waves in the jugular venous pulse occur in

    A pulmonary stenosis
    B left ventricular hypertrophy
    C tricuspid regurgitation
    D atrial fibrillation
    E constrictive pericarditis

23. Indications for thrombolytic therapy in suspected acute myocardial infarction include

    A new-onset right bundle branch block
    B dominant R waves and ST depression in leads V1–V3
    C ST-segment depression >0.2 mV in two adjacent chest leads or >0.1 mV in two or more limb leads
    D presentation more than 24 hours after onset of chest pain with continuing pain and ECG evidence of an evolving infarct
    E following successful traumatic cardiopulmonary resuscitation (CPR)

24. Management of the acute coronary syndrome includes

    A oxygen
    B morphine
    C adrenaline
    D glyceryl trinitrate
    E aspirin

25. Management of atrial fibrillation may include

    A atropine
    B verapamil
    C propranolol
    D flecainide
    E DC cardioversion

26. Wolff–Parkinson–White Syndrome

    A is associated with an accessory pathway (bundle of Kent) connecting to the ventricle some distance from the bundle of His.
    B is associated with a delta wave during the SVT
    C is best treated with intravenous adenosine
    D is associated with a delta wave which lengthens the PR interval
    E may be treated with intravenous verapamil

27. Relative contraindications to streptokinase treatment following a myocardial infarction include

    A pregnancy
    B treatment with streptokinase in the previous three months
    C hypotension
    D total hip replacement operation in the previous three weeks
    E warfarin treatment with an INR of 3.0

28. The following statements regarding the hypothalamus are correct

    A Lesions of the posterior hypothalamus result in obesity.
    B Bilateral lesions of the ventromedial nucleus result in loss of appetite.
    C The posterior hypothalamus responds to excessive heat by vasodilation of skin vessels.
    D Hypothalamic lesions result in loss of short-term memory.
    E It produces oxytocin.

29. Obstructive sleep apnoea

    A may be caused by a redundant uvula
    B may be caused by deviation of the nasal septal cartilage
    C may be caused by lymphoid hyperplasia in a child
    D is best investigated by polysomnography
    E is associated with cessation of respiratory effort for a period of time

30. Guillain–Barré syndrome may be associated with

    A normal CSF
    B facial nerve palsy
    C distal muscle wasting
    D easily elicited sensory deficits
    E infectious mononucleosis

31. Clinical features of carotid artery stenosis include

    A amaurosis fugax
    B hemiparesis
    C hemisensory loss
    D transient global amnesia
    E palpable bruit

32. Characteristic features of sciatica include

    A increased ankle jerk reflex
    B weakness of plantar flexion
    C decreased sensation over the dorsum of the foot
    D pain radiating into the buttock
    E pain radiating down front of the leg

33. Side-effects of lithium carbonate include

    A polydipsia
    B fine tremor
    C exacerbation of psoriasis
    D hyperthyroidism
    E hyperkalaemia

34. Features of Horner's syndrome include

    A ptosis
    B miosis
    C contralateral anhidrosis
    D enophthalmos
    E ophthalmoplegia

35. Common signs of schizophrenia include

    A auditory hallucinations
    B flat affect
    C delusions of persecution
    D pressured speech
    E social withdrawal

36. Cardinal features of dementia include

    A hallucinations
    B emotional blunting
    C dysphasia
    D depression
    E delusions of persecution

37. Symptoms of anxiety may include

   A globus hystericus
   B loss of appetite
   C palpitations
   D tetany
   E headache

38. Risk factors for successful suicide attempts include

   A unemployment
   B female gender
   C age under 40
   D mental illness
   E alcohol abuse

39. Characteristic features of mania include

   A visual hallucinations
   B impaired insight
   C poverty of speech
   D flight of ideas
   E grandiose delusions

40. The following features would favour a diagnosis of delirium rather than dementia

   A dysphasia
   B speech perseveration
   C emotional blunting
   D visual hallucinations
   E restlessness

41. A positive direct antiglobulin Coombs' test occurs in

   A methylodopa-induced haemolytic anaemia
   B cord blood of infants with haemolytic disease of the newborn
   C paroxysmal cold haemoglobinuria
   D infectious mononucleosis
   E type IV delayed hypersensitivity reaction

42. Diverticular disease of the colon may be complicated by

   A acute toxic dilatation
   B bowel perforation
   C carcinoma of the colon
   D pneumaturia
   E severe rectal bleeding

43. Pseudomembranous colitis

   A is associated with overgrowth of Clostridium difficile
   B is more often sensitive to metronidazole than vancomycin
   C is not cured until the toxin of the causative organism has been eliminated
   D is a hazard of prolonged antibiotic therapy
   E should not be treated until antibiotic sensitivities are known

44. Late complications of acute pancreatitis include

   A pseudocyst
   B hyperglycaemia
   C abscess
   D hypocalcaemia
   E acute renal failure

45. Causes of neutropenia include

   A kala-azar
   B SLE
   C Churg–Strauss syndrome
   D brucellosis
   E splenomegaly in rheumatoid arthritis (Felty's syndrome)

46. Causes of acute pancreatitis include

   A azathioprine
   B mumps
   C polyarteritis nodosa
   D hypercalcaemia
   E hyperlipidaemia

47. Clinical features of thyrotoxicosis include

   A pretibial myxoedema
   B menorrhagia
   C lid lag
   D thyroid bruit
   E ophthalmoplegia

48. Clinical features of Cushing's syndrome include

   A hirsutism
   B menorrhagia
   C osteomalacia
   D hypertension
   E keloid wound healing

49. A false low total serum thyroxine concentration may be associated with

    A amiodarone
    B aspirin
    C chronic ethanol intake
    D oral contraceptive pill
    E phenytoin

50. Causes of short stature include

    A adult coeliac disease
    B homocystinuria
    C hypopituitarism
    D hypothyroidism
    E primary hypogonadism

51. The following drugs are safe to use in mild renal impairment

    A erythromycin
    B flucloxacillin
    C fluoxetine
    D metformin
    E neomycin

52. Plasma renin

    A converts angiotensinogen to angiotensin I
    B is produced in the juxta glomerular apparatus
    C levels increase in response to excess dietary sodium
    D acts on the distal renal tubule to reabsorb sodium and water from the urine
    E is released by increased intravascular volume

53. Extra-articular features of rheumatoid arthritis include

    A nail pitting
    B skin ulceration
    C keratoconjunctivitis sicca
    D fibrosing alveolitis
    E carpal tunnel syndrome

54. Recognised features of osteoarthritis include

    A subchondral sclerosis
    B Osler's nodes
    C osteophyte formation
    D extensor deformities
    E fibrillation of cartilage

55. HLA-B8 and HLA-DR3 are associated with

    A juvenile rheumatoid arthritis
    B chronic active hepatitis
    C SLE
    D Behçet's disease
    E polycystic kidney disease

56. Conditions associated with monoarthritis include

    A gonorrhoea
    B osteoarthritis
    C rheumatoid arthritis
    D pseudogout
    E Henoch–Schönlein purpura

57. Nail abnormalities are recognised features in

    A chlamydia infection
    B cirrhosis
    C hypoalbuminaemia
    D primary hyperparathyroidism
    E psoriasis

58. Trigger factors for psoriasis include

    A beta-haemolytic streptococcal throat infection
    B emotional stress
    C exposure to sunlight
    D repeated mechanical skin trauma
    E smoking

59. Pruritus is associated with

    A dermatitis herpetiformis
    B hypothyroidism
    C lichen planus
    D pernicious anaemia
    E polycythaemia rubra vera

60. Palmar erythema may be associated with

    A SLE
    B pregnancy
    C rheumatoid arthritis
    D thyrotoxicosis
    E polycythaemia rubra vera

Answers to Paper Three MCQs

Criterion Referencing Marks

*   – 25–50% of candidates expected to get correct
**   – 50–75% of candidates expected to get correct
*** – 75–100% of candidates expected to get correct

The notional PASS MARK is 228/300 or 76%

1. TTFFT *** Loss of lacrimation is tested by the Schirmer's test and implies a lesion proximal to the greater superficial petrosal nerve. The forehead muscles are spared in UMN lesions.

2. TTTFF ***

3. FTFFT *** Helicobacter pylori is a Gram-negative organism and may go unnoticed. Most patients with duodenal ulcers are found to harbour this organism.

4. FFTTT **

5. TFTTF *** Turner's syndrome is 45, XO. Waardenburg's syndrome is an autosomal dominant condition associated with a white forelock, heterochromia and sensorineural hearing loss. Edwards' syndrome is 47, +18. Patau's syndrome is 47, +13. Treacher–Collins syndrome is an autosomal dominant condition characterised by microtia, hypoplasia of the malar, maxilla and mandible bones, resulting in a conductive hearing loss.

6. TTFFT * Case-control studies are retrospective. Cohort studies are prospective and generate incidence data.

7. FFFTT ** The median is the middle score of an ordered frequency distribution. The mode is the value that occurs most commonly in a distribution. The mean is the arithmetic average obtained by adding all the scores and dividing by the number of scores. A positively skewed distribution is one in which the mean is greater than the median.

8. TTFTF *** Hepatitis C virus is associated with an increased risk of hepatocellular carcinoma and over 50% develop chronic hepatitis.

9. TTTTT ***

10. FTTTF ** Complications of mycoplasma pneumoniae include Coombs' positive haemolytic anaemia, erythema multiforme, GI symptoms (D's & V's), Guillain–Barré syndrome, thrombocytic purpura, and bullous myringitis.

11. TTFTF ** According to the BNF, chloroquine once weekly is recommended prophylaxis in North Africa and the Middle East. Elsewhere chloroquine is recommended in conjunction with proguanil hydrochloride 200 mg once daily. Doxycyline is recommended in chloroquine-resistant areas such as Oceania. Benign malaria is associated with Plasmodium vivax.

12. TFTTF **

13. FTTTF *** Female gender is a good prognostic factor.

14. FFFFF *** Aspirin poisoning is associated with tinnitus, vomiting and hyperventilation.

15. FTFFT ** Blood groups A, B and AB are associated with an increased risk of thrombosis on the combined oral contraceptive pill. It is not proven to cause weight gain and is prescribed for PMT.

16. FFFFT ** Hereditary angioedema results from a complement deficience. The rest except for Wiskott–Aldrich syndrome are associated with defective phagocytes.

17. FTFFT *** Adrenaline has both α and β-adrenergic activity and may be administered via the tracheal tube.

18. TFTFT ** Concomitant verapamil (calcium-channel blocker) and beta-blockers may result in asystole, severe hypotension and heart failure. Warfarin effects are enhanced by antibacterials such as chloramphenicol, ciprofloxacin, cotrimoxazole, metronidazole, erythromycin, clarythromycin and neomycin. Metronidazole inhibits the metabolism of phenytoin and phenobarbital enhances the metabolism of metronidazole. Metoclopramide enhances the absorption of analgesics such as paracetamol and is used concomitantly in the treatment of migraines. Thiazides enhance the risk of lithium toxicity, less so with the use of loop diuretics such as frusemide.

19. FTTTT ** Amiodarone increases the duration of the action potential.

20. FFTTT *** Verapamil reduces conduction through the AV node and is negatively inotropic.

21. FTTFT *** Hypothyroidism is associated with acute pericarditis.

22. TTFFF ** Other causes of a large "a" wave include pulmonary hypertension and tricuspid stenosis.

23. FTFFF *** Thrombolytic therapy is used for new-onset LBBB and ST-segment elevation >0.2 mV in two adjacent leads or >0.1 mV in two or more limb leads. Presentation may be between 12 and 24 hours after onset of chest pain with continuing pain +/– ECG evidence of an evolving infarct. Traumatic CPR is a relative contraindication to the use of thrombolytic therapy.

24. TTFTT ***

25. FFTTT *** Amiodarone and heparin may also be used to treat AF.

26. TFTFT ** The delta wave shortens the PR interval.

27. TTFTT ** Relative contraindications to streptokinase therapy include treatment with streptokinase over 4 days prior (associated with the development of antibodies); traumatic CPR; major surgery less than 4 weeks prior; anticoagulant therapy with an INR >2.5; known bleeding disorder; recent internal bleeding within 4 weeks; active peptic ulcer disease; pregnancy; and severe uncontrolled hypertension.

28. TFFFF *. A lesion of the lateral hypothalamus is associated with loss of appetite. A lesion of the posterior hypothalamus is associated with obesity. The anterior hypothalamus responds to excessive heat. Lesions of the hippocampus affect short-term memory. The posterior pituitary gland produces oxytocin.

29. TTTTF *** Central sleep apnoea is associated with the cessation of respiratory efforts. Obstructive sleep apnoea is associated with increased respiratory efforts to overcome the obstruction to the nasopharynx.

30. TTFFT *** Guillain–Barré is associated with proximal and not distal muscle wasting.

31. TTTFF ***

32. FTFTT ** Sciatica is associated with decreased ankle jerk reflex and decreased sensation over the sole of the foot.

33. TTTFF *** Side-effects of lithium include hypothyroidism and hypokalaemia.

34. TTFTF *** Ipsilateral anhidrosis (lack of facial sweating) is associated with Horner's syndrome (due to a sympathetic lesion).

35. TTTFT *** Schizophrenics demonstrate poverty of speech.

36. TTTTF **

37. TFTTT ***

38. TFFTT *** Older, unemployed men are at higher risk of successful suicide. Other risk factors include mental and physical illnesses and drug and alcohol abuse.

39. FTFTT *** Mania is associated with pressured speech and euphoria.

40. FTFFF *** Dysphasia and emotional blunting are features of dementia. Visual hallucinations and restlessness feature in both conditions.

41. TTTTF ** Coombs' test is an example of a Type II (cytotoxic) hypersensitivity reaction.

42. FTFTT ***

43. TFTTF *** Pseudomembranous colitis should be treated promptly prior to drug sensitivities.

44. TFTFF *** Hyperglycaemia, hypocalcaemia and acute renal failure are all early complications of acute pancreatitis.

45. TTFTT *** Churg–Strauss syndrome is associated with eosinophilia.

46. TTTFT ***

47. TFTTT ***

48. TFFTF *** Cushing's syndrome is associated with amenorrhoea, osteoporosis and impaired wound healing.

49. TTFTF * The oral contraceptive pill and pregnancy are both associated with falsely elevated total serum T4.

50. FFTTF ** Homocystinuria, thyrotoxicosis and Marfan's syndrome are associated with tall stature.

51. TTTFF * According to the BNF metformin and neomycin should be avoided in renal impairment.

52. TTFFF *** Plasma renin responds to decreased intravascular volume. Concentrations decrease in response to excess sodium. Aldosterone and not renin acts on the distal renal tubule.

53. FTTTT ***

54. TFTFT *** Osteoarthritis is associated with Heberden's nodes and fixed flexion deformities.

55. FTTFF ** Juvenile RA is associated with HLA-B27. Behçet's and polycystic kidney disease are associated with HLA-B5.

56. FTFTF ** Gonorrhoea, rheumatoid arthritis, Henoch–Schönlein purpura, Sjogren's, SLE, viral infections, inflammatory bowel disease and drug reactions are associated with polyarthritis. Septic arthritis, trauma, gout, spondylarthritides, osteoarthritis and TB arthritis are associated with monoarthritis.

57. FTTFT ***

58. TTFTT **

59. TFTFT ***

60. FTTTT ***

In these questions candidates must select one answer only

Questions

1. A 40-year-old forester presents with a peculiar rash that started as a small papule. The rash now consists of multiple red rings up to 5 cm in diameter with raised borders and faded centres. He also complains of headache, fever and lymphadenopathy. The MOST likely diagnosis is

   A mycoplasma infection
   B Borrelia burgdorferi infection (Lyme disease)
   C tuberculosis
   D rheumatic fever
   E pityriasis rosea

2. Metronidazole is indicated for the treatment of all the following infections EXCEPT

   A bacterial vaginosis
   B trichomoniasis
   C giardia lamblia
   D clostridium difficile
   E chlamydia trachomatis

3. A 22-year-old HIV-positive Ugandan man presents with hypopigmented anaesthetic annular lesions with raised erythematous rims and painful nodules on his left forearm and legs. On examination a thickened ulnar nerve is palpated at the left elbow and running into the lesions. He is also noted to have multiple transverse white lines on his fingernails. The MOST likely diagnosis is

   A leprosy
   B syphilis
   C leptospirosis
   D tuberculosis
   E sarcoidosis

4. The MOST useful investigation would be

A complement fixation test
B skin smear for AFB
C biopsy of thickened nerve
D Kveim test
E FTA and VDRL

5. A 40-year-old woman presents with dysuria and urinary incontinence. She has a history of having passed urinary calculi in the past. Her urine is noted to have an alkaline pH. The MOST likely organism is

A Escherischia coli
B Proteus mirabilis
C Atypical Streptococci
D Pseudomonas aeruginosa
E Klebsiella sp.

6. A 20-year-old HIV-positive man presents with fever and meningism. CSF shows

Pressure	250 mm H20
WBCs	200/mm^3
Predom. Cells	lymphocytes
Glucose	33% plasma level
Protein	5 g/L

Possible diagnoses include the following EXCEPT

A cryptococcal meningitis
B coccidioides meningitis
C tuberculous meningitis
D carcinomatous meningitis
E histoplasma meningitis

7. The following statements regarding human parvovirus B19 are correct EXCEPT

A may cause aplastic crises in patients with sickle cell disease
B produces erythema infectiosum
C produces hand foot and mouth disease
D causes chronic anaemia in immunocompromised patients
E may cause aplastic crises in patients with hereditary spherocytosis

8. A 70-year-old man, who lives alone and is self-caring, presents with weakness in his lower legs and muscle pain. On examination he has loose teeth and is noted to have ecchymoses of the lower limbs. He suffers from rheumatoid arthritis, which greatly limits his mobility. The MOST likely diagnosis is

A folate deficiency
B scurvy
C iron deficiency
D thiamine deficiency
E vitamin B$_{12}$ deficiency

9. A 35-year-old African woman is found to have a Hb of 6 g/dL. She is a vegetarian and has a history of uterine fibroids. Her blood film reveals microcytic, hypochromic red blood cells and a few target cells. The MOST likely diagnosis is

A thalassaemia trait
B iron-deficiency anaemia
C sickle cell disease
D anaemia of chronic disease
E sideroblastic anaemia

10. A 25-year-old woman presents with a single, non-tender enlarged cervical lymph node. She also complains of fever and night sweats. Lymph node biopsy reveals infiltration with histiocytes and lymphocytes and the presence of cells with bi-lobed mirror-image nuclei. The MOST likely diagnosis is

A non-Hodgkin's lymphoma
B Hodgkin's lymphoma
C sarcoidosis
D acute lymphoblastic leukaemia
E tuberculosis

11. A 70-year-old edentulous man presented with bruising and bone and joint pain. On examination he has nail splinters haemorrhages. The back of his legs are covered with haemorrhages into the muscles and ecchymoses. X-ray of his legs show subperiosteal haemorrhages. The MOST useful diagnostic text is

A capillary fragility test
B blood cultures
C bone marrow aspirate
D folic acid level
E platelet ascorbic acid levels

12. The following statements regarding amiodarone are correct EXCEPT

    A Amiodarone is a class Ib anti-arrhythmic drug.
    B It acts to prolong the action potential.
    C It does not affect sodium transport through the membrane.
    D It is arrhythmogenic if given with drugs that prolong the QT interval.
    E It is associated with abnormalities of thyroid function.

13. The absolute contraindication to thrombolytic therapy IS

    A INR >2.5
    B recent head trauma
    C suspected aortic dissection
    D known bleeding disorder
    E pregnancy

14. Which one of the following drugs CANNOT be administered via the tracheal route?

    A adrenaline
    B atropine
    C amiodarone
    D lignocaine
    E naloxone

15. The following cardiac drugs are correctly paired with their corresponding indications for use EXCEPT

    A amiodarone – haemodynamically stable ventricular tachycardia
    B lignocaine – first-line drug for refractory ventricular fibrillation
    C magnesium sulphate – torsades de pointes
    D adenosine – paroxysmal supraventricular tachycardia
    E verapamil – supraventricular tachycardia

16. The following statements regarding digoxin are true EXCEPT

    A It increases vagal tone.
    B It decreases sympathetic drive.
    C It increases conduction velocity in the Purkinje fibres.
    D It is less effective than amiodarone in acute atrial fibrillation.
    E It prolongs AV node refractory period.

17. The following statements regarding tricyclic antidepressant poisoning are correct EXCEPT

    A It may be treated by activated charcoal.
    B Oral diazepam is usually adequate to sedate delirious patients.
    C The use of anti-arrhythmics is strongly advised.
    D It is associated with dilated pupils and urinary retention.
    E It is associated with hypothermia and hyper-reflexia.

18. Recommended treatment for salicylate poisoning includes all of the following EXCEPT

    A forced alkaline diuresis
    B haemodialysis
    C activated charcoal by mouth
    D urinary alkalinisation with sodium bicarbonate
    E charcoal haemoperfusion

19. A 60-year-old woman presents with progressive forgetfulness and mood changes. She has a shuffling gait. Her brain CT scan shows cortical atrophy and enlarged ventricles. Histology shows senile plaques and neurofibrillary tangles. The MOST appropriate treatment is

    A levodopa in combination with a dopa-decarboxylase inhibitor
    B donepezil
    C tetrabenazine
    D diazepam
    E thiamine

20. The following statements regarding anti-epileptic drugs are correct EXCEPT

    A Carbamazepine is the drug of choice for absence seizures.
    B Sodium valproate is the drug of choice for myoclonic seizures.
    C Lamotrigine is the drug of choice for seizures associated with Lennox–Gastaut syndrome.
    D Carbamazepine may be used as prophylaxis of bipolar disorder unresponsive to lithium.
    E Carbamazepine is associated with Stevens–Johnson syndrome.

21. A 50-year-old man complains of difficulty in hearing and dyspnoea. He is noted to have a nasal septal perforation and a blood pressure of 140/90. His urinalysis shows red cells, protein and casts. The chest x-ray reveals opacities. The MOST appropriate treatment for the condition described is

A rifampicin, isoniazid, pyrazinamide and ethambutol
B cyclophosphamide
C plasmaphoresis
D penicillin
E short-course of prednisolone

22. The following clinical manifestations are associated with sarcoidosis EXCEPT

A finger clubbing
B lupus pernio
C pulmonary fibrosis
D erythema nodosum
E facial nerve palsy

23. A 40-year-old man presents with a painful and swollen right knee joint. The synovial fluid is opaque and bloody with no white cells or crystals. Possible diagnoses include the following EXCEPT

A Charcot joint
B haemophilia
C osteosarcoma
D aseptic necrosis
E chondrocalcinosis

24. A 40-year-old woman complains of difficulty placing an object on a high shelf and of combing her hair. She also has trouble climbing and descending the stairs. She adds that she has difficulty swallowing food. She is sensitive to the cold and does not smoke or drink alcohol. On examination, she has weakness in the muscles of the neck, shoulder girdle, hips and thighs. Deep tendon reflexes are mildly reduced. Her blood tests reveal elevated creatinine kinase, AST, ALT and LDH. Electromyography shows fibrillation potentials. The MOST likely diagnosis is

A Eaton–Lambert syndrome
B amyotophic lateral sclerosis
C dystrophia myotonica
D polymyositis
E myasthenia gravis

25. A 60-year-old woman presents with morning stiffness in both knees and pain worse at the end of the day. On examination the knees are swollen and warm to the touch with a flexion deformity and limitation of movement. X-ray shows narrowing of the joint spaces, osteophytes at the margin of the joints and sclerosis of the underlying bone. The MOST likely diagnosis is

A rheumatoid arthritis
B osteoarthritis
C gout
D infective arthritis
E polymyalgia rheumatica

26. Recognised treatment for this condition include all of the following EXCEPT

A total knee replacement
B NSAIDs
C penicillamine
D intra-articular corticosteroid
E physiotherapy

27. The following statements regarding acute myocardial infarction are correct EXCEPT

A A lateral infarction is usually seen in leads V5–6 and/or leads I and aVL.
B An inferior infarction results often from a lesion in the right coronary artery.
C Patients with an anterior infarction benefit more from thrombolysis and treatment with ACE inhibitors than at other sites.
D Acute coronary syndrome is defined as infarction with new LBBB.
E Initial management for acute MI should include morphine, oxygen, GTN and aspirin.

28. The following statements regarding electrocardiography are correct EXCEPT

A Electrodes should be placed over muscle not bone to minimise electrical interference.
B A completely straight line usually does not indicate asystole.
C Standard paper speed is 25 mm/sec.
D Pulseless electrical activity signifies the absence of cardiac output in the presence of any form of electrical activity.
E Fine ventricular fibrillation (VF) has a worse prognosis than coarse VF.

29. The following statements regarding the internal jugular vein (IJV) are correct EXCEPT

A It initially lies in front of the carotid artery.
B As it descends in the neck it lies lateral to the common carotid artery.
C On the right it joins the subclavian vein to form the brachiocephalic vein.
D IX–XII cranial nerves and the phrenic nerve are closely related to the IJV in the neck.
E The site of insertion for central vein cannulation is the apex of the triangle formed by the 2 heads of the sternomastoid muscle.

30. A 50-year-old man presents with bradycardia of 30 beats/min. His systolic blood pressure is 80. He has a productive pink frothy cough and basal crackles on auscultation. ECG confirms sinus bradycardia and inferior myocardial infarction. There has been no satisfactory response to an initial 500 µg IV of atropine. The NEXT most appropriate management for this man would be

A repeat atropine to maximum 3 mg
B adrenaline 2–10 µg/min as an IV bolus
C isoprenaline IV infusion
D transcutaneous pacing on the T wave
E transvenous pacing

31. A 70-year-old man presents to the outpatient clinic with a 2-month history of worsening breathlessness and chest pain on exertion. On examination you note an ejection systolic murmur in the aortic region, an early high-pitched diastolic murmur of the left lower sternal edge and pulsus biferiens. The MOST likely diagnosis is

A infective endocarditis
B left atrial myxoma
C rheumatic aortic valvular disease
D impending myocardial infarction
E congestive cardiac failure

32. The MOST useful investigation would be

A 12-lead electrocardiogram
B echocardiogram
C cardiac catheterisation
D cardiac isoenzymes and troponin
E chest x-ray

33. A 55-year-old smoker with a history of chronic productive cough presents to Casualty breathless and drowsy. On examination he is centrally cyanosed with a raised JVP and a palpable liver. There is a pansystolic murmur at the lower left sternal border. No abnormality is heard in the lungs. The MOST likely diagnosis is

   A infective endocarditis
   B cor pulmonale
   C ventricular septal defect
   D exacerbation of chronic bronchitis
   E emphysema

34. The MOST useful diagnostic investigation is

   A arterial blood gas
   B 12-lead electrocardiogram
   C lung function tests
   D chest x-ray
   E sputum examination

35. The MOST appropriate treatment is

   A continuous oxygen therapy
   B frusemide
   C salbutamol inhaler
   D oral prednisolone 30 mg od
   E amoxycillin 500 mg o tds

36. The inspired oxygen content using a bag-valve-mask with oxygen but no reservoir IS

   A 16%
   B 21%
   C 40%
   D 50%
   E 85%

37. The following are recognised features of obstructive sleep apnoea EXCEPT

   A hypnagogic hallucinations
   B impotence
   C morning headaches
   D nightmares
   E daydreaming

38. A 20-year-old arrives to Casualty with marked dyspnoea; he suffers from asthma. On examination respiratory rate 24/min and pulse 105/min. The peak flow is 60% of predicted. The MOST appropriate management would be

A treat in casualty with nebulised salbutamol 5 mg and repeat peak flow in 30 mins.
B arrange immediate hospital admission and treat with IV hydrocortisone 200 mg
C arrange immediate hospital admission, administer oxygen 40–60%, nebulised salbutamol and oral prednisolone 30–60 mg
D arrange immediate hospital admission, administer oxygen-driven nebuliser and give slow IV aminophyline 250 mg
E treat in casualty with oral prednisolone 30–60 mg and repeat peak flow in 30 mins.

39. An 18-year-old man presents with fever, stridor and trismus. His breathing becomes laboured with use of accessory muscles. He becomes cyanosed with a respiratory rate of 35, despite oxygen by face mask. He had initially presented to his GP a few days ago with a sore throat. He takes salbutamol inhaler for his asthma. The MOST appropriate management in Casualty would be:

A endotracheal intubation
B needle cricothyroidotomy
C tracheostomy
D IV hydrocortisone
E nasopharyngeal airway

40. The MOST likely diagnosis is

A glandular fever
B streptococcal throat infection
C acute asthma attack
D angioneurotic oedema
E tetanus

41. A 60-year-old priest presents with cough, dyspnoea, dull chest pain and vague epigastric pain. On examination the left chest shows diminished expansion, stony dull percussion note and absent breath sounds. There is aegophony at the apex. The mediastium is shifted to the right. The chest x-ray confirms a unilateral pleural effusion. The MOST useful investigation would be

A CT chest
B sputum for culture and sensitivity
C aspiration of pleural effusion
D bronchoscopy
E V/Q scan

42. A pleural tap shows

Specific gravity	1.020
Total protein	40 g/L
LDH	300 IU (70–250 IU/L)
Amylase	300 Somogyi U/dL (0–180 Somogyi U/dL)

Possible diagnoses include the following EXCEPT

A acute pancreatitis
B pancreatic pseudocyst
C lung cancer
D oesophageal rupture
E tuberculosis

43. Examples of physiological shunting include all of the following EXCEPT

A pulmonary fibrosis
B pulmonary embolism
C pulmonary oedema
D COPD
E atelectasis

44. A 30-year-old female involved in a road traffic accident is brought by ambulance to Casualty. She is noted to have bruising over the mastoid process and periorbital haematoma. On otoscopic examination she has bleeding behind the tympanic membrane. The MOST likely diagnosis is

A extradural haematoma
B subdural haematoma
C basal skull fracture
D depressed occipital skull fracture
E intracerebral haemorrhage

45. A 60-year-old man presents with rigidity and bradykinesia. He has an ataxic gait. On examination he has postural hypotension without compensatory tachycardia and his pupils are asymmetric. The MOST likely diagnosis is

A multi-infarct dementia
B Alzheimer's disease
C Friedreich's ataxia
D Parkinson's disease
E Shy–Drager syndrome

46. The following pathological findings and diseases are correctly paired EXCEPT

   A Lewy bodies – Parkinson's disease
   B plaques of demyelination – multiple sclerosis
   C neurofibrillary tangles – Alzheimer's disease
   D Negri bodies – rabies
   E sulphur granules – variant CJD (related to BSE)

47. A 40-year-old man is brought to Casualty in a comatose state. Useful initial investigations include all of the following EXCEPT

   A serum glucose
   B serum calcium
   C arterial blood gases
   D full blood count
   E blood alcohol level

48. On examination he is noted to have constricted pupils and depressed respirations. The MOST appropriate management would be:

   A head CT scan
   B naloxone 0.4–1.2 mg IV stat
   C flumazenil 200 mcg IV over 15 sec.
   D doxapram IV
   E dantrolene 1mg/kg IV

49. A 20-year-old man is found unconscious after a night of binge drinking. There is no evidence of physical trauma. On examination he has alcohol on his breath and a bitten tongue. Blood pressure 110/80 and pulse 80/min. The pupils are small, equal and responsive to light. On removal of his clothes, his trousers are noted to be soiled with urine. The MOST likely explanation for his unconscious state is

   A hypoglycaemic coma
   B alcoholic overdose
   C post-ictal phase of an epileptic seizure
   D subarachnoid haemorrhage
   E narcotic drug overdose

50. A 40-year-old pedestrian has been struck by a speeding car. He is brought to Casualty wearing a pneumatic antishock garment for an extensive open avulsion injury to his pelvis. He is intubated with fluids running via 2 large-bore intravenous cannulas. His blood pressure is 120/80. The pelvis is grossly distorted. The NEXT most appropriate management as a casualty officer would be

A take blood for full blood count, type and cross 6 units, urea and electrolytes and commence O negative blood infusion

B cut away the man's clothing and perform a thorough physical examination

C insert a Foley catheter after a digital rectal examination to exclude a high riding prostate

D perform a brief neurological examination

E notify the orthopaedic surgeons to apply an external fixator

51. A 25-year-old man presents with unilateral eye pain of acute onset, blurring of vision, photophobia, lacrimation, red eye and a small pupil. The pain is exacerbated on testing of accommodation and the pupil is seen to constrict. The MOST likely diagnosis is

A acute closed angle glaucoma

B acute iritis

C acute conjunctivitis

D ulcerative keratitis

E subconjunctival haemorrhage

52. The MOST appropriate management for this patient is

A lie the patient flat and refer urgently to ophthalmologist

B sit the patient upright and refer urgently to ophthalmologist

C place the patient at a 45 degree angle and refer urgently to ophthalmologist

D prescribe IV diamox and refer urgently to ophthalmologist

E arrange for urgent Doppler scan of the carotid

53. A 20-year-old man presents with persistent eye irritation. He explains that he is sensitive to light, has noted worsening vision and complains of aching eyes. He also complains of morning stiffness in his back. The MOST likely diagnosis is

A keratitis

B uveitis

C viral conjunctivitis

D episcleritis

E choroiditis

54. The MOST useful investigation for this man would be

    A lumbar and pelvic spine x-ray
    B Kveim test
    C HIV test
    D Mantoux test
    E rheumatoid factor

55. A 70-year-old long-sighted woman presents to Casualty at midnight with vomiting that began three hours earlier and slightly worsening vision. The eyeball is rock-hard on palpation. The conjunctiva is injected. The MOST appropriate management for this patient is

    A dilate pupil with tropicamide to examine the retina
    B give antiemetic and refer to ophthamologist in the morning
    C oral prednisolone
    D give antiemetic and IV diamox and refer to on-call ophthalmologist urgently
    E prescribe fucithalmic ointment bd

56. The following statements regarding Good Medical Practice (GMC code) are correct EXCEPT

    A You must provide the necessary care to alleviate pain and distress whether or not curative treatment is possible.
    B You may end a professional relationship with a patient if he or she makes a complaint about you or your team.
    C In an emergency, wherever it may arise, you must offer anyone at risk the assistance you could reasonably be expected to provide.
    D You must respond constructively to the outcome of appraisals of your performance.
    E You must take part in adverse event recognition and reporting to help reduce risk to patients.

57. Diagnostic features of post-traumatic stress disorder include all of the following EXCEPT

    A autonomic arousal
    B recurrent, obtrusive thoughts
    C symptoms of anxiety
    D memory impairment
    E loss of orientation

58. Diagnostic features of panic disorder include all of the following EXCEPT

A dizziness
B feelings of unreality
C fear of insanity
D fear of leaving home
E choking sensations

59. Diagnostic features of mania include all of the following EXCEPT

A labile mood
B rapid speech
C loss of inhibitions
D overeating
E grandiosity

60. The following statements regarding GOOD MEDICAL PRACTICE are correct EXCEPT

A You may end professional relationships with patients if they have persistently acted inconsiderately.
B You must assist the coroner by offering all relevant information to an inquest.
C You are not entitled to remain silent if your evidence may lead to criminal proceedings being taken against you.
D If you have grounds to believe that a doctor may be putting patients at risk, you must give an honest explanation of your concerns to a medical director.
E You must not refuse to treat a patient because you may be putting yourself at risk.

61. A 45-year-old woman presents with pruritis, pale stools and dark urine. On examination she has finger clubbing and hepatosplenomegaly. Her blood tests reveal a normal bilirubin, elevated alkaline phosphatase and low T4. The MOST certain way to confirm the diagnosis is by

A anti-mitochondrial antibody
B liver biopsy
C ERCP
D CT scan of the abdomen
E hepatitis A, B and C serology

62. The MOST likely diagnosis is

A viral hepatitis
B chronic autoimmune active hepatitis
C suppurative cholangiohepatitis
D primary sclerosing cholangitis
E primary biliary cirrhosis

63. A 60-year-old man presents with increasing abdominal girth. On examination you elicit shifting dullness. The MOST useful investigation would be

A CT scan of the abdomen
B ascitic fluid tap
C ultrasound of the abdomen
D chest x-ray
E blood for FBC, urea and electrolytes, LFTS and amylase

64. A 65-year-old man presents with a 2-month history of vague lower abdominal pain, alternating diarrhoea and constipation and 4kg weight loss. He has passes a small amount of dark red blood per rectum. He is anaemic. The MOST useful investigation is

A flexible sigmoidoscopy
B barium enema
C CT scan of abdomen
D abdominal ultrasound
E selective mesenteric angiograpy

65. A 45-year-old woman presents with pruritis and jaundice. She complains of dry eyes and mouth. The MOST discriminating investigation would be

A mitochrondial antibodies
B antinuclear antibody
C serum bilirubin and liver function tests
D HBs antigen
E smooth muscle antibody

66. Causes of air under the diaphragm include all of the following EXCEPT

A Crohn's disease
B perforated duodenal ulcer
C pleuroperitoneal fistula
D laparoscopy
E ruptured ectopic pregnancy

67. A 50-year-old man presents in shock with rigors and a temperature of 40°C. He is jaundiced and is tender on palpation of the liver, which is felt 5 cm below the costal margin. Dark concentrated urine is noted upon Foley catheter insertion. The MOST likely diagnosis is

A ascending cholangitis
B gallstone ileus
C hepatitis
D primary sclerosing cholangitis
E acute cholecystitis

68. A 54-year-old diabetic man presents with fever, and a painful and swollen right lower leg. On examination, the pulses are absent distally, the foot cold and subcutaneous crepitus is present. The MOST useful investigation is

A x-ray of the leg
B Doppler ultrasound
C arteriogram
D blood cultures
E venogram

69. The MOST likely diagnosis is

A osteomyelitis
B gas gangrene
C chronic ischaemia of the leg
D deep venous thrombosis
E acute ischaemia of the leg

70. A 66-year-old woman presents in a coma. Temperature 35°C, pulse 50 and BP 140/80. On examination she has a goitre and few basal rales in the chest. Her deep tendon reflexes are not brisk. Her medication is thyroxine, bendrofluazide, and omeprazole. Blood results:

Plasma sodium	129 mmol/L
Plasma potassium	3.6 mmol/L
Plasma urea	10 mmol/L
Plasma creatinine	130 μmol/L
Plasma glucose	3 mmol/L

The MOST likely underlying diagnosis is

A renal failure
B Addisonian crisis
C hypoglycaemia
D congestive heart failure
E myxoedema

71. A 55-year-old man complains of generalised weakness for the past month. He also complains of excessive thirst and frequent micturition. Blood results:

Urine glucose	negative
Urine nitrate	negative
Serum creatinine	140 μmol/L
Serum urea	10 mmol/L
Serum calcium	3.5 mmol/L
Serum phosphate	1 mmol/L
Serum alkaline phosphatase	200 IU/L (30–300 IU/L)
Serum albumin	45 g/L

These findings are consistent with all of the following diseases EXCEPT

A primary hyperparathyroidism
B sarcoidosis
C multiple myeloma
D thyrotoxicosis
E bone metastases

72. The following are useful investigations to establish the diagnosis EXCEPT

A full blood count
B chest x-ray
C ESR
D parathyroid hormone
E magnesium

73. His chest x-ray reveals bilateral hilar lymphadenopathy. The MOST likely diagnosis is

A primary hyperparathyroidism
B sarcoidosis
C multiple myeloma
D thyrotoxicosis
E bone metastases

74. A 25-year-old woman presents to the outpatient clinic with a neck swelling. On examination the swelling moves upward with protrusion of the tongue. The MOST likely diagnosis is

A thyroid goitre
B cystic hygroma
C thyroglossal cyst
D branchial cyst
E thyroid malignancy

75. The following are recognised causes of respiratory alkalosis EXCEPT

   A high altitude
   B salicylates
   C pulmonary emboli
   D right to left pulmonary shunt
   E flail chest

76. The following are recognised causes of mixed metabolic alkalosis and respiratory alkalosis EXCEPT

   A pregnancy and vomiting
   B hepatic failure and diuretics
   C chronic respiratory failure and mechanical ventilation
   D Gram-negative septicaemia
   E massive blood transfusion

77. Causes of hypercalcaemia associated with decreased parathyroid hormone include all of the following EXCEPT

   A Addison's disease
   B thyrotoxicosis
   C recovery from acute tubular necrosis
   D Paget's disease
   E immobilisation

78. The BEST initial investigation of female infertility is

   A transvaginal ultrasound
   B chromosomal karyotype
   C prolactin level
   D demonstration of rise of progesterone during the luteal phase
   E diagnostic laparoscopy

79. A 20-year-old woman presents with secondary amenorrhoea. The urine pregnancy test is negative. Her basal plasma prolactin level is 350 mU/L (60–390). She is given a progestogen challenge and has withdrawal bleeding. The MOST likely diagnosis is:

   A polycystic ovarian disease
   B prolactinoma
   C gonadal dysgenesis
   D chronic anovulation with oestrogen absent
   E Mullerian agenesis

80. Causes of hyperprolactinaemia include all of the following EXCEPT

    A hyperthyroidism
    B sarcoidosis
    C metoclopramide
    D pituitary tumour
    E pregnancy

81. The following statements regarding parathyroid hormone (PTH) are correct EXCEPT

    A Pseudohypoparathyroidism is due to failure of target cells to respond to PTH.
    B Secondary hyperparathyroidism is associated with raised PTH appropriate to low calcium.
    C Secondary hyperparathyroidism usually occurs following neck surgery.
    D The most common cause of primary hyperparathyroidism is a single benign adenoma.
    E Primary hyperparathyroidism is associated with MEN type I.

82. A 60-year-old man presents to Casualty with painless profuse haematuria for the past 2 days. On examination BP 90/50 and pulse 105/min. Blood results:

White cell count	5×10^9/L
Hb	6 gm/dL
Platelets	150×10^9/L
Serum creatinine	300 µmol/L
Serum urea	20 mmol/L

    Following resuscitation, the patient is no longer bleeding. The MOST useful investigation would be

    A cystoscopy
    B intravenous pyelogram
    C ultrasound of the kidneys, bladder and prostate
    D pelvic CT scan
    E retrograde urography

83. A 42-year-old woman presents to Casualty with right-sided colicky loin pain and nausea for the past 3 hours. She cannot keep still because of the pain. She has a history of recurrent cystitis. Temperature 36.5°C, BP 110/60 and pulse 60/min. Urinalysis shows microscopic haematuria. The MOST likely diagnosis is

    A pelvic inflammatory disease
    B acute pyelonephritis
    C acute appendicitis
    D nephrolithiasis
    E ectopic pregnancy

84. The MOST useful initial diagnostic investigation is

    A serum urea and electrolytes
    B urine β-HCG
    C plain KUB film
    D pelvic ultrasound
    E IV urogram

85. While in Casualty the patient develops fever and rigors. The MOST likely complication that has occurred is

    A ruptured ectopic pregnancy
    B exacerbation of pelvic inflammatory disease
    C ruptured appendix
    D acute pyelonephritis
    E septicaemia

86. A 70-year-old man presents to the outpatient clinic complaining of difficulty urinating and dribbling. On abdominal examination he has a distended bladder that reaches the umbilicus. He also complains of back pain. The NEXT most appropriate step would be

    A take blood for serum urea, creatinine and electrolytes
    B take blood for PSA and acid phosphatase
    C perform a digital rectal examination
    D insert a Foley catheter
    E MSU for urinalysis and MC&S

87. Causes of proximal renal tubular acidosis include all of the following EXCEPT

    A Wilson's disease
    B carbonic anhydrase inhibitors
    C multiple myeloma
    D hyperparathyroidism
    E chronic active hepatitis

88. A 40-year-old man presents with fever, backache and acute obstructive renal failure. His Hb is 9 gm/dL, and he has a raised ESR. IV urogram shows dilated ureters with medial deviation of the ureters. The MOST likely diagnosis is

    A ureteric stone obstruction
    B obstructive megaureter
    C retroperitoneal fibrosis
    D pelvi-ureteric junction obstruction
    E obstructive nephropathy secondary to malignancy

89. A 30-year-old woman with Crohn's disease presents with left flank pain and microscopic haematuria. She admits she doesn't drink enough water. She smokes, drinks wine and loves chocolates. X-ray shows a radioopaque left renal calculus. The MOST likely aetiology is

    A hypercalciuria
    B hyperoxaluria
    C hyperuricaemia
    D cystinuria
    E hyperuricosuria

90. Dietary recommendations you would make for her include avoidance of all of the following EXCEPT

    A spinach
    B rhubarb
    C chocolate
    D tomatoes
    E tea

91. A 25-year-old man presents with nonpruritic white spots on his trunk. On examination there are multiple sharply demarcated round depigmented macules of up to 2 cm in size. On gentle scratching, a delicate scaling is noted. There is no associated lymphadenopathy. There is no family history of depigmentation. Organisms are seen on direct microscopy. The MOST likely diagnosis is

    A psoriasis
    B pinta
    C leprosy
    D vitiligo
    E pityriasis versicolor alba

92. White nails are associated with all of the following conditions EXCEPT

    A psoriasis
    B renal failure
    C arsenic poisoning
    D cytotoxic drug therapy
    E cirrhosis

93. A 45-year-old woman with diabetes presents with shiny waxy erythematous plaques on her shins with yellowish skin and telangiectasia. The MOST likely diagnosis is

A pretibial myxoedema
B pyoderma gangrenosum
C psoriasis
D erythema nodosum
E necrobiosis lipoidica

94. A 30-year-old man presents with fever, arthralgia and a palmar rash. On examination he has oral vesicles and circular lesions on his palms. The MOST likely diagnosis is

A Stevens–Johnson syndrome
B Behçet's syndrome
C herpes simplex
D syphilis
E hand-foot-mouth disease

95. Photodermatitis is a complication of all of the following drugs EXCEPT

A demeclocycline
B frusemide
C oral contraceptives
D nalidixic acid
E barbiturates

96. Alopecia is a recognised complication of all of the following EXCEPT

A withdrawal from oral contraceptives
B heparin
C ethionamide
D cytotoxic drugs
E sulfonamides

97. A 16-year-old girl is brought to Casualty by her mother. She complains of persistent and worsening dull right-sided lower abdominal pain and spotting of blood per vagina. The mother insists her daughter is a virgin. On examination temperature 36.5°C, BP 90/50 and pulse 120/min. The lower abdomen is rigid with rebound tenderness in the right iliac fossa. Her period is overdue. The MOST appropriate management following resuscitation is

A ask to speak to the girl in private, and obtain confidential information from her as to whether she has been sexually-active. If so, perform a urinanalysis, urine β-HCG pregnancy test and pelvic exam with triple swabs.

B arrange for urgent transvaginal ultrasound to exclude ectopic pregnancy

C accept that the daughter is a virgin, omit a pelvic internal exam and take a low vaginal swab to exclude infection

D arrange for pelvic ultrasound to exclude ectopic pregnancy and acute appendicitis

E inform the mother that you are performing a urine pregnancy test in the best interests of her daughter to exclude possibility of a miscarriage or ectopic pregnancy

98. A 30-year-old woman presents with a spiking temperature and a foul-smelling vaginal discharge 24 hours after delivery of her baby. She has been sexually active with her partner throughout the pregnancy. The MOST likely organism is

A group A streptococcus
B group B streptococcus
C chlamydia trachomatis
D gardnerella vaginalis
E neisseria gonorrhoea

99. Neisseria gonorrhoea may infect all of the following areas EXCEPT

A vagina
B rectum
C pharynx
D conjunctiva
E urethra

100. The following statements regarding Chlamydia trachomatis are correct EXCEPT

A It is the commonest cause of non-gonococcal urethritis.
B It is more often symptomatic in women.
C It causes Reiter's syndrome.
D It is treated with doxycycline.
E It causes perihepatitis.

Answers to Paper Three BOFs

Criterion Referencing Marks

*   – 25–50% of candidates expected to get correct
**   – 50–75% of candidates expected to get correct
***   – 75–100% of candidates expected to get correct

The notional PASS MARK is 76%

1. B **

2. E ***

3. A **

4. C **

5. B ***

6. D ** Carcinomatous meningitis is associated with the presence of mononuclear cells.

7. C ** Hand foot and mouth disease is caused by Coxsackie A16 virus.

8. B ***

9. B ***

10. B ***

11. E ***

12. A *** Amidarone is a class III anti-arrhythmic drug.

13. C ***

14. C *

15. B *** Lignocaine is a second-line drug for treatment of refractory ventricular fibrillation.

16. C *** Digoxin decreases the conduction velocity in the Purkinje fibres.

17. C ** Arrhythmias associated with TCA poisoning should respond to correction of hypoxia and acidosis.

18. A ** Forced alkaline diuresis is no longer recommended by the British National Formulary (BNF).

19. B ***

20. A *** Ethosuximide and sodium valproate are the drugs of choice in the treatment of absence seizures.

21. B ***

22. A ***

23. D **

24. D **

25. B ***

26. C *** Penicillamine is a form of treatment for rheumatoid arthritis.

27. D *** Acute coronary syndrome also includes non-Q-wave MI, unstable angina and Q-wave MI.

28. A ***

29. A ** The internal jugular vein initially lies behind the carotid artery in the neck.

30. A *** Adrenaline is given by IV infusion and not by bolus. Pacing is performed on the R wave and not the T wave. The latter would kill the patient!

31. C ***

32. B ***

33. B ***

34. A *** ECG changes in cor pulmonale include P pulmonale, RAD, RVH and inverted T waves in V1-4. The chest x-ray and sputum may be normal. Lung function tests will show airflow obstruction. Arterial blood gases will confirm hypoxia and show degree of hypercapnia which is important in guiding management.

35. A ***

36. D **

37. E *** OSA is associated with carbon dioxide retention and may manifest as morning headaches.

38. A ***

39. B * Needle cricothyroidotomy may be necessary as an emergency procedure in casualty. The leading cause of death from glandular fever (infectious mononucleosis) is failed endotracheal intubation! Bear in mind that the patient has jaw trismus! Needle cricothyroidotomy will buy time for tracheostomy by an ENT surgeon in theatre.

40. A ***

41. C ***

42. E *** All the options produce pleural exudates but tuberculosis is the only one not associated with increase in amylyase.

43. B ** Pulmonary embolism is a cause of physiological dead space.

44. C **

45. E **

46. E *** Sulphur granules are associated with actinomycosis.

47. E ***

48. B ***

49. C ***

50. A ***

51. B *

52. A *

53. B **

54. A **

55. D * This patient has acute angle closure glaucoma. Pupils dilate at dusk which close off the angle. Visual loss can result from use of dilators! IV diamox (acetazolamide) is recommended to reduce pressures. This patient has 6–8 hours before impending visual loss and requires urgent referral.

56. B ***

57. E **

58. C ***

59. D ***

60. C ***

61. B ***

62. E ***

63. B ***

64. A ***

65. A ***

66. E ***

67. A *** The patient exhibits Charcot's triad.

68. A **

69. A **

70. E ***

71. E ** Bone metastases are usually associated with low albumin and increased alkaline phosphatase.

72. E ***

73. B ***

74. C ***

75. E *** Flail chest is associated with respiratory acidosis.

76. D ** Gram-negative sepsis is associated with mixed metabolic acidosis and respiratory alkalosis.

77. C **

78. D **

79. A **

80. A *** Hyperprolactinaemia may occur in hypothyroidism not hyperthyroidism.

81. C *** Primary hypoparathyroidism is associated with neck surgery.

82. B **

83. D ***

84. C ***

85. D ***

86. C ***

87. D ** Hyperparathyroidism is associated with distal renal tubular acidosis.

88. C ***

89. B **

90. D **

91. E * The organism is the yeast Pityrosporum orbiculare.

92. A **

93. E ***

94. A ***

95. E **

96. E **

97. A **

98. B **

99. A * Neisseria gonorrhoea affects columnar epithelium. The vagina is composed of squamous epithelium. This explains why the endocervix and not the vagina is swabbed for the presence of the organism.

100. B *** Chlamydia is often asymptomatic in women.

MRCP Paper Four MCQs

Questions

1. An ulnar nerve lesion at the elbow would result in

   A claw hand deformity
   B loss of flexion at the distal interphalangeal joint of the little finger
   C loss of the supinator reflex
   D inability to open the fist
   E Froment's sign (overcompensation by the flexor pollicis longus)

2. Injury to the common peroneal nerve at the neck of the fibula results in

   A inability to invert the foot
   B inability to dorsiflex the great toe
   C loss of ankle jerk reflex
   D loss of sensation on the sole of the foot
   E weakness of plantar flexion

3. A lesion affecting the lateral cord of the brachial plexus gives rise to

   A paralysis of the biceps brachii
   B inability to flex the dorsal interphalangeal (DIP) of the index finger
   C weak supination
   D loss of palmar sweating
   E wasting of the intrinsic small muscles of the hand

4. Pupillary light reflex depends upon an intact

   A optic nerve
   B oculomotor nerve
   C ophthalmic nerve
   D midbrain
   E occipital cortex

5. The following are causes of metabolic acidosis

   A starvation
   B uraemia
   C metformin
   D paracetamol poisoning
   E hyperaldosteronism

6. The following statements regarding cystic fibrosis are correct

A The abnormal gene is on chromosome 7.
B Pseudomonas cepacea is associated with rapidly progressive lung disease.
C Steatorrhoea is a characteristic feature.
D Cells are relatively impermeable to chloride.
E Allergic bronchopulmonary aspergillosis is a recognised feature.

7. The following statements are correct

A The alternate hypothesis represents lack of difference between samples and population data.
B A Type II error is an error of commission, i.e. detecting a difference when none exists.
C A Type I error is failing to recognise a true experimental result.
D The null hypothesis indicates true experimental effect and that the obtained values are unlikely to be due to random fluctuations among samples.
E The power of a statistical test is the ability of a test to detect a true difference.

8. The following statements are correct

A The correlation coefficient ranges from negative one to positive one.
B A positive correlation is one in which both variables increase.
C A correlation coefficient of zero indicates independence i.e. a change in one variable is not associated with a change in the other variable.
D The coefficient of determination is the square of the correlation coefficient.
E Correlation and regression assume that a linear relationship does not exist between the two variables X and Y.

9. The following statements are correct

A Prevalence rate per 1000 is the number of new cases of a disease occurring in a population during a specified period of time divided by the number of people exposed to the risk of developing disease during that time multiplied by 1000.
B Incidence rate per 1000 is the number of cases of a disease present in a population at a specified time divided by the number of people in the population at a specified time multiplied by 1000.
C Specificity is true positives (TP) divided by all those who have the disease (TP+False negatives (FN)).
D Sensitivity is true negatives (TN) divided by all those who do not have the disease (TN+False positives (FP)).
E P=0.05 means that the result of a statistical test is deemed significant if there is only a 1 in 20 chance that the result occurred by chance alone.

10. Recognised features of homocystinuria include

    A autosomal recessive inheritance
    B upward lens dislocation
    C osteomalacia
    D mental retardation
    E morphological resemblance to Marfan's syndrome

11. Down's syndrome is associated with

    A duodenal atresia
    B lymphoblastic leukaemia
    C simian palmar crease
    D macroglossia
    E atrial septal defect

12. The HLA-B27 antigen is characteristically found in

    A Behçet's syndrome
    B Reiter's syndrome
    C Crohn's disease
    D Sjogren's syndrome
    E psoriatic arthropathy

13. Giardiasis

    A is often asymptomatic
    B is treated with metronidazole
    C can be excluded by negative stool microscopy for cysts and
      trophozoites
    D may result in GI malabsorption and steatorrhoea
    E is caused by a flagellated protozoon that is transmitted by faeces

14. Characteristic features of osteosarcoma include

    A around the hip being the commonest site
    B new bone formation
    C highest incidence among 25–35-year-olds
    D spread by the bloodstream
    E chemotherapy improves the prognosis

15. Causes of megaloblastic anaemia include

    A thalassaemia
    B zidovudine (AZT)
    C alcohol
    D myxoedema
    E leukaemia

16. Recognised features of von Willebrand's disease (Factor VIII deficiency) include

    A autosomal recessive inheritance
    B abnormal platelet count
    C prolonged clotting time
    D deficient platelet aggregation in response to ristocetin
    E haemarthroses

17. Causes of hyperprolactinaemia include

    A metoclopramide
    B chronic renal failure
    C breast-feeding
    D hyperthyroidism
    E amenorrhoea

18. Complications of steroid therapy include

    A diabetes insipidus
    B osteoporosis
    C hypertensive crisis immediately postoperative
    D depression
    E proximal myopathy

19. Absolute contraindications to the combined oral contraceptive pill include

    A body mass index (BMI) >30
    B migraine with focal aura
    C successfully treated malignant melanoma
    D diabetic non-smoker
    E sickle cell trait

20. Non-steroidal anti-inflammatory drugs

    A selectively inhibit cyclo-oxygenase
    B are contra-indicated in asthmatics
    C may lead to renal papillary necrosis
    D when given by rectal suppository avoid gastric side-effects
    E are contra-indicated in the presence of suspected cerebrovascular bleeding

21. Characteristic features of acute salicylate poisoning include

A sweating
B vomiting
C tinnitus
D hypoventilation
E confusion

22. Contraindications to the use of propranolol include

A second degree AV block
B bronchospasm
C uncontrolled cardiac failure
D phaeochromocytoma
E myasthenia gravis

23. Recognised side-effects of metronidazole include

A peripheral neuropathy
B erythema nodosum
C renal impairment
D disulfiram-like reaction with alcohol
E jaundice

24. The following drugs are contraindicated in the post-natal period if the mother opts to breast-feed

A ethinyloestradiol + levonorgestrel (microgynon)
B norethisterone (micronor)
C medroxy progesterone acetate i.m (depo-provera)
D diclofenac
E amoxycillin

25. Major criteria for the diagnosis of rheumatic fever include

A complete heart block
B erythema multiforme
C shortened PR interval
D subcutaneous nodules
E pericarditis

26. Features of acute cardiac tamponade include

A pulsus paradoxus
B increased jugular venous pressure on inspiration
C hypertension
D muffled heart sounds
E cardiogenic shock

27. Patients with the following conditions are at significant risk for endocarditis

A aortic stenosis
B atrial septal defect
C bicuspid aortic valve
D persistent ductus arteriosus
E mitral valve prolapse

28. Digoxin is contraindicated in

A congestive heart failure
B supraventricular tachycardia
C intermittent complete heart block
D pregnancy
E recent myocardial infarction

29. Mitral stenosis is associated with

A a diastolic murmur that increases in intensity with exercise
B a murmur that decreases in intensity with age
C a higher risk of infective endocarditis
D atrial fibrillation
E rheumatoid arthritis

30. Recognised associations of sleep apnoea include

A cor pulmonale
B Wolff–Parkinson–White (WPW) syndrome
C deviated nasal septum
D high alcohol intake
E obesity

31. The peak expiratory flow rate is

A correlated well with vital capacity
B increased in emphysema
C the maximum rate of flow at any time during forced expiration
D dependent on effort
E used to monitor the response of asthma to treatment

32. Causes of bronchiectasis include

A allergic bronchopulmonary aspergillosis
B hypogammaglobulinaemia
C post measles infection
D cystic fibrosis
E asthma

33. Features of the hyperventilation syndrome include

A dysphagia
B dyspnoea
C rotatory vertigo
D chest pain
E carpopedal spasm

34. Causes of lower motor neurone facial nerve palsy include

A acute suppurative otitis media
B cholesteatoma
C parotid adenoid cystic tumour
D posterior inferior cerebellar artery syndrome
E pseudobulbar palsy

35. Features of petit mal epilepsy (absence attacks) include

A brief pauses lasting 10 seconds
B 3/second Hz spike and wave EEG activity
C ethosuximide and sodium valproate as drugs of choice
D partial (focal) seizures
E loss of consciousness

36. Features of motor neurone disease include

A extraocular muscle involvement
B dysphagia
C altered sensation
D fasciculation
E positive Babinski sign

37. Drugs known to aggravate epilepsy include

A co-proxamol (paracetamol + dextropropoxyphene)
B withdrawal of benzodiazepines
C chlorpromazine
D imipramine
E cocaine

38. Characteristic EEG abnormalities of diagnostic value are seen in

A petit mal seizures
B temporal lobe epilepsy
C hemiplegia
D trigeminal neuralgia
E sleep apnoea

39. Characteristic elements of alcohol dependence syndrome include

    A subjective awareness of a compulsion to drink
    B increased tolerance to alcohol
    C relief from or avoidance of withdrawal symptoms by further drinking
    D broadening of the drinking repertoire
    E delirium tremens

40. Toxic serum lithium concentrations may cause

    A renal failure
    B hypertension
    C convulsions
    D hyperkalaemia
    E hyper-reflexia of the limbs

41. The following statements regarding sleeping sickness are correct

    A It is transmitted by a sandfly.
    B The lymph glands are tender and rubbery.
    C It is associated with choreiform movements.
    D It is associated with apathy and a mask-like facies.
    E Pentamidine is used when CNS involvement occurs.

42. In Crohns' disease

    A sulphasalazine improves ileal disease
    B prednisolone improves the prognosis
    C tall stature may be a feature
    D mouth ulcers may be a manifestation
    E metronidazole may improve colonic disease

43. Gallbladder distension may be associated with carcinoma of the

    A common bile duct
    B duodenum
    C tail of the pancreas
    D ampulla of Vater
    E common hepatic duct

44. The following statements regarding ulcerative colitis are correct

    A The risk for colonic carcinoma increases after 5 years.
    B Salazopyrin may cause male infertility.
    C Skip lesions are a recognised feature.
    D The rectum is always involved.
    E Persistent severe mucosal dysplasia is an indication for surgery.

45. Causes of paralytic ileus include

    A acute pancreatitis
    B hyperkalaemia
    C retroperitoneal haematoma
    D spinal injury
    E biliary colic

46. Duodenal ulcer

    A occurs more commonly in females
    B classically produces pain following a meal
    C pain is worse during the day
    D has an increasing incidence in the UK
    E should be treated in the first instance with antihelicobacter triple
       therapy

47. The following statements regarding yellow fever are correct

    A It is a tick-borne disease.
    B It is associated with hepatic midzonal necrosis and hytalin deposits
       (councilman bodies).
    C High fever and bradycardia occur early in the illness.
    D Jaundice occurs in the convalescent phase.
    E Treatment is with penicillin.

48. Symptoms of hypoglycaemia include

    A transient hemiplegia
    B sweating
    C postural hypotension
    D hyperventilation
    E personality change

49. Diabetes mellitus may be associated with

    A papilloedema
    B ptosis
    C absent ankle jerk reflex
    D pruritis vulvae
    E malignant otitis externa

50. The following conditions and clinical features are correctly paired

    A pityriasis rosea – the herald patch
    B Microsporum audouini – fluoresce bluish-white on ultraviolet Wood's light
    C dermatitis herpetiformis – itchy polymorphic rash over flexor surfaces
    D Stevens–Johnson syndrome – erythema marginatum
    E multiple myeloma – pyoderma gangrenosum

51. Characteristic features of Klinefelter's syndrome include

    A XYY karyotype
    B enlarged testes
    C low IQ
    D shortened life span
    E gynaecomastia

52. Features of Cushing's syndrome due to ectopic ACTH production include

    A hyperkalaemia
    B pigmentation
    C weight gain
    D clinical symptoms of greater prominence than biochemical abnormalities
    E failure of urinary or plasma cortisol suppression on high-dose dexamethasone test

53. The following drugs should be avoided in severe liver disease

    A mefenamic acid
    B nifedipine
    C pyrazinamide
    D labetalol
    E promethazine (phenergan)

54. The following organisms and conditions are correctly paired

    A Mycobacterium tuberculosis – lupus pernio
    B Staphylococcus aureus – erysipelas
    C Streptococcal infection – impetigo
    D Corynebacterium minutissimum – erythrasma
    E Herpes simplex virus I – erythema multiforme

55. Characteristic features of Type I renal tubular acidosis include

    A osteoporosis
    B renal calculi
    C a urine pH <6 in the presence of acidaemia
    D hyperkalaemia
    E constipation

56. Type 4 renal tubular acidosis is associated with

    A amyloidosis
    B amiloride
    C Addison's disease
    D hypokalaemia and acidic urine
    E hyporeninaemic hypoaldosteronism

57. Wegener's granulomatosis is associated with

    A rapidly progressive glomerulonephritis
    B raised titre of c (cytoplasmic) ANCA in 95% of cases
    C raised titre of p (perinuclear) ANCA in 95% of cases
    D nasal crusting and discharge
    E haemoptysis

58. Osteoarthritis may be a complication of

    A rheumatoid arthritis
    B osteochondritis of the hip (Perthes disease)
    C rheumatic fever
    D haemophilia
    E septic arthritis

59. Characteristic features of Reiter's syndrome include

    A aortic incompetence
    B circinate balanitis
    C episcleritis
    D pompholyx
    E relapsing arthritis

60. Gum abnormalities are found with

    A Addison's disease
    B acute myeloid leukaemia
    C beri-beri
    D Vincent's angina
    E ethosuximide

Answers to Paper Four MCQs

Criterion Referencing Marks

*   – 25–50% of candidates expected to get correct
**   – 50–75% of candidates expected to get correct
*** – 75–100% of candidates expected to get correct

The notional PASS MARK is 222/300 or 74%

1. FTFFF * Claw hand deformity and positive Froment's sign (pinching a piece of paper between the thumb and index finger leads to flexion of the DIP) are seen with low lesions to the ulnar nerve i.e. at the wrist. Loss of supinator jerk and inability to open a fist are associated with radial nerve injury. Paralysis of the small muscles of the hand does occur but the lateral two lumbricals and the thenar muscles are spared. High injuries (at the elbow) result in paralysis of flexor carpi ulnaris and the ulnar aspect of flexor digitorum profundus.

2. FTFFF * Injury to the common peroneal nerve results in an inability to dorsiflex and to evert the ankle. The tibial nerve supplies sensation to the sole of the foot. Injury to S1 results in loss of ankle jerk reflex.

3. TTFFF * A lesion affecting the lateral cord of the brachial plexus would result in weak pronation. A lesion affecting the medial cord of the brachial plexus would result in wasting of the intrinsic small muscles of the hand, weakness of the long finger flexors and an ipsilateral Horner's syndrome.

4. TTFTF ***

5. TTTTF *** Other causes of metabolic acidosis include drug poisoning (salicylate, alcohol, paraldehyde), ketoacidosis (diabetes, alcohol), and lactic acidosis (severe exercise, shock, hypoxia, biguanide drugs, acute liver failure, leukaemia, lymphoma).

6. TTFTT ***

7. FFFFT * The definitions of Type I and Type II errors are reversed. The definitions of null and alternate hypotheses are reversed.

8. TTTTF * Correlation and regression assume that a linear relationship does exist.

9. FFFFT ** The definitions for prevalence and incidence have been reversed. The definitions for sensitivity and specificity have also been reversed.

10. TFFTT *** Homocystinuria is associated with downward lens dislocation and osteoporosis not osteomalacia.

11. TTTFT ***Other associations with Down's syndrome include hypothyroidism, VSD, patent ductus, Brushfield iris spots, and widely spaced 1st and 2nd toe digits.

12. FTFFT ** Behçet's syndrome is associated with HLA-B5 and HLA-DR5. Sjogren's syndrome is associated with HLA-B8 and HLA-DRw3. HLA-B27 is most commonly found in ankylosing spondylitis.

13. TTFTT **

14. FTFTF ** Osteosarcoma has a predilection for the knee. The highest incidence is among 15–25-year-olds.

15. FTFTT ***

16. FFFTF *** Von Willebrand's disease is an autosomal dominant inherited disease of factor VIII deficiency. It is associated with a normal clotting time and normal platelet count. The bleeding time is prolonged.

17. TTTFT *** Hyperprolactinaemia is associated with hypothyroidism.

18. FTFTT *** Adrenal insufficiency is a complication of steroid therapy and may result in precipitous hypotension in the intraoperative and immediate postoperative period.

19. FTFFF ** Well-controlled diabetes in a young non-smoker is classified as WHO2 or relative risk. She can be commenced on a low-dose combined oral contraceptive pill. A diabetic who smokes is classified as WHO4, an absolute contraindication. Sickle cell disease and not trait is an absolute contraindication. Only migraine associated with a focal aura or treated with ergotamine is an absolute contraindication.

20. TTTFT ***

21. TTTFT *** Salicylate poisoning is associated with hyperventilation.

22. TTTTF *** Propranolol is not contraindicated in myasthenia gravis and can be used with caution.

23. TFFTT ** Side-effects of metronidazole also include erythema multiforme and hepatitis.

24. TFFFF * Microgynon is a form of combined oral contraceptive pill, which contains oestrogen and therefore is contraindicated in breast-feeding. Micronor is a progestogen-only pill (pop) and is safe during breast-feeding. The pop is usually prescribed 3 weeks post delivery when the mother is fertile. Precautions should be taken for a further week. Depo-provera is a form of progestogen-only injectable and is safely administered 6 weeks post delivery.

25. TFFTT *** Rheumatic fever is associated with erythema marginatum and prolonged PR interval.

26. TTFTT *** Cardiac tamponade is associated with hypotension, increased JVP and muffled heart sounds (Beck's triad).

27. FFTTT ** Conditions associated with increased risk of endocarditis include mitral valve prolapse, ventricular septal defect, patent ductus arteriosus, congenital and rheumatic heart valve disease, and prosthetic heart valves.

28. FTTFF ** Digoxin is a form of treatment for congestive heart failure. Digoxin may be prescibed but with caution in pregnancy and following a recent MI.

29. TFFTF *** Mitral stenosis is most commonly due to rheumatic heart disease.

30. TFTTT ***

31. FFTTT *** The PEFR is decreased in emphysema. It correlates well with FEV$_1$.

32. TTTTF ***

33. FTFTT *** Features of the hyperventilation syndrome also include panic attacks, palpitations, sweating, dizziness, paresthesiae and choking sensation. Diagnosis is made on provocation test. Management involves reassurance, relaxation exercises and rebreathing into a paper bag.

34. TTTTF **

35. TTTFF ** Absence attacks are examples of generalised seizures.

36. FTFTT *** MND never affects sensation or extra-ocular movements associated with cranial nerves III, IV and VI.

37. FTTTT ** Phenothiazines and tricyclic antidepressants are associated with aggravation of epilepsy and should be administered with caution in epileptics.

38. TFFFF ***

39. TTTFT ** The alcohol dependence syndrome includes all of the mentioned elements as well as primacy of drinking over other activities and rapid reinstatement of syndrome on drinking after a period of abstinence.

40. TFTFT ** Severe lithium toxicity is also associated with hypokalaemia, hypotension, circulatory collapse, coma and death.

41. FFTTF * Sleeping sickness is caused by the bite of the tsetse fly. Manifestations of African sleeping sickness or trypanosomiasis include discrete non-tender, rubbery lymph nodes, hepatosplenomegaly, mask-like facies, day-time somnolence; later signs include hyperaesthesia over the ulnar nerve (Kerandel's sign), choreiform movements, fits and coma. Myocarditis occurs in the acute Rhodesian form of sleeping sickness. Prognosis is good if treatment begins before brain invasion.

42. FFFTT *** Sulfasalazine does not help ileal disease. Prednisolone does not alter the prognosis. Crohn's disease is associated with growth retardation in children.

43. TTFTF *** Gallbladder distension may be associated with carcinoma of the head of the pancreas and not the tail.

44. FTFTT *** Increased risk of colonic cancer is seen at 10 years. The colon is always affected in continuity.

45. TFTTF *** Paralytic ileus is associated with hypokalaemia.

46. FFFFT *** Duodenal ulcers present more commonly in men, at night and are associated with Helicobacter pylori infection. Food relieves the pain. Triple therapy with a proton pump inhibitor (omeprazole or lansoprazole), clarithromycin and amoxicillin or metronidazole is advocated to eradicate H. pylori which is found in cases of relapse.

47. FTTTF * Yellow fever is a mosquito-borne infection. Aedesaegyptic is the Vector. Treatment is supportive.

48. TTFFT ***

49. FTTTT ***

50. TFFFT *** Microsporum audouini fluoresces green. Bluish-white light is the normal colour from a Wood's light. Dermatitis herpetiformis is associated with a rash over the extensor surfaces and is associated with coeliac disease. Stevens–Johnson syndrome is associated with erythema multiforme.

51. FFTFT *** Klinefelter's syndrome is either XXY or XXYY karytope. Features include small, firm testes, low IQ, tall stature, gynaecomastia, and a normal life span.

52. FTFFT *** The classical ectopic ACTH syndrome is associated with hypokalaemia, muscle weakness, short history, pigmentation, weight loss, diabetes, elevated plasma bicarbonate levels and a plasma ACTH >200 ng/L. Chest x-ray, whole lung and mediastinal CT scans are recommended to exclude bronchial carcinoma.

53. TFTTF ** NSAIDs should be avoided according to the British National Formulary (BNF). Nifedipine and heparin may be administered but at reduced dosages. Other drugs listed in the BNF that must be avoided in severe hepatic disease include carbamazepine, phenytoin, phenobarbital, metformin, and rifampicin. Promethazine (Phenergan) is the safest sedative.

54. FFFTT *** TB is associated with lupus vulgaris. Staphylococcal infection is associated with impetigo and streptococcal with erysipelas. HSV1 is the most common cause of erythema multiforme.

55. FTFFT ** Type I RTA is associated with osteomalacia and a urine pH >6 in the presence of acidaemia.

56. TTTFT ** Type IV RTA is associated with hyperkalaemia and acidic urine.

57. TTFTT ** Only 20–40% will have raised p-ANCA titres.

58. TTFTT ***

59. TTFFT *** Features of Reiter's syndrome also include keratoderma blenorrhagica, conjunctivitis and painful uveitis.

60. TTFTT ***

MRCP Paper Four BOFs

In these questions candidates must select one answer only

Questions

1. Toxoplasma gondii infection in patients with AIDS may present with any of the following EXCEPT

   A chorioretinitis
   B seizures
   C myocarditis
   D hepatitis
   E encephalitis

2. The organism responsible for gas gangrene IS

   A clostridium difficile
   B clostridium perfringens
   C clostridium tetanus
   D klebsiella sp.
   E pseudomonas aeruginosa

3. The following diseases are associated with the Ebstein–Barr virus EXCEPT

   A craniopharyngioma
   B Burkitt's lymphoma
   C sinonasal tumours
   D glandular fever
   E Hodgkin's lymphoma

4. Shock is associated with all of the following changes EXCEPT

   A increased protein metabolism
   B decreased free fatty acids
   C increased liver glycogenolysis
   D increased uric acid
   E increased lactic production

5. A 60-year-old man presents with dementia. He has a past history of a subarachnoid haemorrhage. He is noted to suffer from urinary incontinence and apraxia. He walks with an unsteady gait. The MOST likely diagnosis is

   A lacunar infarct
   B normal pressure hydrocephalus
   C Creutzfeldt–Jakob syndrome
   D lateral medullary syndrome
   E progressive multifocal leuco-encephalopathy

6. Typhoid fever is associated with all of the following EXCEPT

   A bowel perforation
   B splenomegaly
   C ulceration of Peyer's patches
   D non-blanching maculopapular rash
   E osteomyelitis

7. A 20-year-old man who has travelled recently to India presents with unexplained fever for 5 days. You suspect typhoid fever. The MOST appropriate investigation would be

   A Widal test measuring serum levels of agglutinins to O and H antigens
   B blood culture
   C marrow culture
   D stool culture
   E urine culture

8. Risk factors predisposing to infection with candidiasis include all of the following EXCEPT

   A poor T-lymphocyte function
   B hyperalimentation
   C diabetes mellitus
   D broad-spectrum antibiotic therapy
   E multiple sex partners

9. The following organisms and disease are correctly paired EXCEPT

   A Streptococcus pyogenes – necrotising fasciitis
   B Staphylococcus epidermidis – toxic shock syndrome
   C Staphylococcus aureus – scalded skin syndrome
   D Staphylococcus aureus – impetigo
   E Streptococcus pyogenes – acute rheumatic fever

10. Haemolytic anaemia is associated with all of the following EXCEPT

    A increased urinary urobilinogen
    B decreased haptoglobin
    C urinary haemosiderin
    D negative direct and characteristically positive indirect Coombs' test
    E increased unconjugated bilirubin

11. A 25-year-old woman self-prescribes vitamins and iron tablets. She presents with acute abdominal pain. She is found to be pancy-topaenic with haemosiderin in her urine and trace haemoglobin. The MOST likely diagnosis is

    A SLE
    B aplastic anaemia
    C myelofibrosis
    D paroxysmal nocturnal haemoglobinuria
    E acute myeloid leukaemia

12. A 20-year-old pregnant black woman presents with fever and joint pains. She has a history of two previous spontaneous early mis-carriages. Her urine reveals 2+ protein. Her blood results show leu-copenia, normocytic normochromic anaemia and thrombocytopaenia. The MOST likely diagnosis is

    A sickle cell disease
    B SLE
    C thalassaemia
    D aplastic anaemia
    E pre-eclampsia

13. The MOST sensitive diagnostic test would be

    A positron emission tomography (PET scan)
    B antibodies to double-stranded DNA
    C positive anti-nuclear antibodies
    D antibody to Ro
    E haemoglobin electrophoresis

14. The MOST useful investigation for her miscarriages would be

    A transvaginal ultrasound
    B chromosome karyotype
    C lupus anticoagulant and anticardiolipin antibody
    D hysterosalpingogram
    E antithrombin III, protein C and S deficiency

15. The following statements regarding haemoglobin are correct EXCEPT

A It consists of 2 globin subunits containing a single haem molecule.
B Haem consists of a porphyrin ring and one atom of iron.
C δ-aminolaevulinic acid (ALA) synthetase is the rate-controlling enzyme in haem synthesis.
D Haem is catabolised to biliverdin.
E Conjugated bilirubin is hydrolysed and the free pigment is reduced to urobilinogen and stercobilinogen in the gut.

16. The following statements regarding transplantation are correct EXCEPT

A The cornea is the MOST commonly transplanted allograft.
B Nephrectomy is required prior to kidney transplant in Goodpasture's syndrome.
C Recent malignancy in the recipient is a contraindication to transplant.
D The MOST common cause of death in patients with transplants is malignancy.
E Reticulum cell sarcoma is common in recipients.

17. A 35-year-old African woman is found to have a Hb of 6g/dL. She is a vegetarian and has a history of uterine fibroids. Her blood film reveals microcytic, hypochromic red blood cells and a few target cells. The MOST likely result of iron studies would be

A low ferritin, high TIBC
B low iron, low TIBC
C raised ferritin, low TIBC
D low serum iron, low TIBC
E normal ferritin, high TIBC

18. The following statements regarding immunosuppressive therapy are correct EXCEPT

A Tacrolimus is a calcineurin agonist.
B Rituximab is used in treatment of chemotherapy-resistant advanced follicular lymphoma.
C Cyclosporin is associated with hypertension in heart transplant patients.
D Gingival hyperplasia is a recognised side-effect of cyclosporin.
E Basiliximab is used for prophylaxis of acute rejection in allogenic renal transplantation.

19. Delayed alloimmunisation by previous blood transfusions is associated with all of the following EXCEPT

A destruction of transfused blood cells by IgM antibodies
B spherocytosis
C reticulocytosis
D positive direct antiglobulin test
E extravascular haemolysis

20. The following statements regarding terfenadine are correct EXCEPT

A Patients are advised to avoid grapefruit juice.
B Ventricular arrhythmias have followed excessive dosage.
C It has been associated with erythema multiforme.
D It should be used cautiously in patients with liver disease.
E It causes marked sedation because it penetrates the blood brain barrier.

21. The following statements regarding octreotide are correct EXCEPT

A It is a somatostatin antagonist.
B It may cause gallstones.
C It may be valuable in cessation of variceal bleeding.
D Abrupt withdrawal is associated with pancreatitis.
E It is indicated for the relief of symptoms associated with carcinoid tumours.

22. A 50-year-old farmer presents with acute shortness of breath, dizziness and severe headache. His skin is red in colour, and he smells of bitter almonds. He mentions that he had been using rodenticides. His condition rapidly deteriorates. The MOST appropriate treatment for him would be

A atropine
B sodium nitrite and sodium thiosulphate
C vitamin K
D dimercaprol
E activated charcoal

23. The following statements regarding tetracyclines are correct EXCEPT

A They are broad-spectrum bacteriocidal antibiotics.
B Demeclocycline may cause reversible nephrogenic diabetes insipidus.
C Absorption is decreased by milk and antacids except for doxycycline.
D They cause dental discolouration and hypoplasia in children.
E They are the drug of choice for non-gonococcal urethritis.

24. The following statements regarding paracetamol poisoning are correct EXCEPT

A Acetylcysteine protects the liver if given within 24 hours of ingestion.
B Activated charcoal is administered if ingestion of 150 mg/kg occurred within the hour.
C It may cause renal tubular necrosis.
D Maximum liver damage occurs 3–4 days following ingestion.
E Patients on enzyme-inducing drugs may develop toxicity at lower plasma-paracetamol concentrations.

25. Hepatic microsomal enzyme-inducing drugs include all of the following EXCEPT

A phenytoin
B carbamazepine
C rifampicin
D alcohol
E warfarin

26. The following statements regarding aminoglycosides are correct EXCEPT

A They are bactericidal antibiotics.
B They are well absorbed from the gut.
C Side-effects include ototoxicity and nephrotoxicity.
D Neomycin is used to reduce colonic bacterial flora in patients with hepatic failure.
E They cross the placenta and may cause fetal VIIIth nerve damage.

27. The following statements regarding antiviral drugs are correct EXCEPT

A Valaciclovir is indicated for treatment of recurrent genital herpes.
B Peripheral neuropathy is a side-effect of didanosine.
C Zidovudine is indicated as monotherapy for prevention of maternal-fetal HIV transmission.
D Parkinsonism is a side-effect of amantadine.
E Ganciclovir is active against cytomegalovirus.

28. The following statements regarding antithyroid drugs are correct EXCEPT

A Carbimazole may induce bone marrow suppression.
B Radioactive sodium iodide is safe in patients with heart disease.
C Propylthiouracil (PTU) does not cross the placenta.
D Carbimazole may be associated with alopecia.
E PTU is associated with aplastic anaemia.

29. A 20-year-old man complains of recurrent lower back pain and stiffness after exercise. He has no morning stiffness. His full blood count and ESR are normal, but he is found to have HLA-B27. X-ray of his lumbar spine and pelvis are normal. The MOST appropriate management would be

A no further investigations and reassure the patient that HLA-B27 can also be found in normal people
B arrange for an ophthalmology referral for slit-lamp examination
C arrange a Kveim test to exclude sarcoidosis
D arrange for barium follow-through
E test for rheumatoid factor

30. Major criteria for the diagnosis of rheumatic fever include all of the following EXCEPT

A polyarthralgia
B chorea
C erythema marginatum
D subcutaneous nodules
E fever

31. The following pairs of HLA antigen and diseases have been correctly paired EXCEPT

A HLA-B27 – Reiter's syndrome
B HLA-B14 and A3 – multiple sclerosis
C HLA-DR4 – rheumatoid arthritis
D HLA-DR3 – idiopathic membranous glomerulonephritis
E HLA-DR2 – Goodpasture's syndrome

32. The following statements regarding juvenile rheumatoid arthritis are correct EXCEPT

A It has a worse prognosis than in adults.
B It is usually associated with a positive rheumatoid factor.
C It may occur before the 16th birthday.
D Clinical features are the same as those in adults.
E It is the MOST commonest type of juvenile chronic arthritis.

33. The following statements regarding urate metabolism are correct EXCEPT

A Thiazide diuretics impair urate secretion in the renal tubules.
B Leukaemia and polycythaemia both increase nucleic acid turnover.
C Allopurinol increases the activity of xanthine oxidase.
D Probenecid acts by inhibition of tubular reabsorption of urate.
E Glucose-6-phosphatase deficiency results in increased urate production.

34. A 38-year-old man presents with painful right wrist and left knee joint a fortnight after an attack of gastroenteritis. Prostatic massage produces a urethral discharge. The synovial fluid shows an abundance of neutrophils and is sterile. The ESR is raised. The MOST likely diagnosis is

    A gonococcal arthritis
    B rheumatoid arthritis
    C salmonella arthritis
    D Reiter's syndrome
    E viral arthritis

35. The MOST appropriate treatment for this man would be

    A amoxycillin
    B non-steroidal anti-inflammatory drug
    C penicillin
    D gold
    E doxycycline

36. The following statements regarding sarcoidosis are correct EXCEPT

    A There is a higher incidence among young black males than caucasians.
    B It MOST commonly involves the mediastinal lymph nodes.
    C A third of cases are associated with erythema nodosum.
    D Scalene node biopsy will be positive in 90% of cases.
    E A negative Kveim test excludes sarcoidosis.

37. The MOST common organism implicated in infective endocarditis is

    A staphylococcus aureus
    B streptococcus viridans
    C streptococcus faecalis
    D staphylococcus epidermidis
    E coxiella burnetii

38. A 25-year-old heroin addict presents with fever and mucosal petechial haemorrhages. On examination he has a pansystolic murmur best heard at the lower sternal edge. He is also noted to have small, flat, erythematous, non-tender macules over the thenar eminence. The MOST likely diagnosis is

    A subacute bacterial endocarditis
    B acute bacterial endocarditis
    C rheumatic heart disease
    D acute rheumatic fever
    E Q fever

39. The following statements regarding verapamil are correct EXCEPT

A It belongs to the class IV anti-arrhythmic drugs.
B It reduces the plateau phase of the action potential.
C It is indicated for supraventricular tachycardia.
D It is contraindicated in the presence of β-blockers.
E It may precipitate digoxin toxicity.

40. The following pulse patterns are correctly matched with their disorders EXCEPT

A pulsus alternans – left ventricular failure
B pulsus paradoxus – cardiac tamponade
C pulsus bisferiens – hypertrophic obstructive cardiomyopathy
D pulsus parvus et tardus (small volume, slow rising) – aortic regurgitation
E dicrotic pulse – dilated cardiomyopathy

41. A 70-year-old man presents with dyspnoea and chest pain. His pulse rate is 120, and he is extremely agitated. His arterial blood gas reveals low arterial oxygen and low CO_2. His ECG shows S wave in I, Q and T waves in III and T wave inversion in leads V1-3. The MOST likely diagnosis is

A myocardial infarction
B pulmonary embolism
C acute pericarditis
D cardiac tamponade
E pneumothorax

42. A 25-year-old healthy male smoker presents with gangrene of the left big toe. There are no signs of external trauma. The MOST likely diagnosis is

A thromboangiitis obliterans (Buerger's disease)
B Raynaud's disease
C gas gangrene
D polyarteritis nodosa
E gout

43. Bilharzia is associated with all of the following EXCEPT

A portal hypertension
B Asian Katayama fever
C haematuria
D type III hypersensitivity reaction
E tropical pulmonary eosinophilia

44. The following statements regarding leukotriene receptor antagonists are correct EXCEPT

    A Churg–Strauss syndrome has been associated with use of these antagonists following the reduction or withdrawal of oral corticosteroid therapy.
    B Zafirlukast is indicated for the prophylaxis of asthma.
    C Montelukast may be used as add-on therapy in severe asthma.
    D They block the effect of cysteinyl leukotrienes in the airways.
    E Montelukast may be used to prevent exercise-induced bronchospasm.

45. Cystic fibrosis is associated with all of the following EXCEPT

    A abnormal gene coding for transmembrane regulating factor protein on chromosome 7
    B allergic bronchopulmonary aspergillosis
    C steatorrhoea
    D chronic infection with pseudomonas pseudomallei
    E diabetes mellitus

46. The following statements regarding lung function tests are correct EXCEPT

    A Total lung capacity = vital capacity + residual volume.
    B A normal transfer factor in the presence of persistently reduced FEV_1 may occur with chronic asthma.
    C In restrictive lung diseases the FEV_1 to FVC ratio is higher than normal.
    D Transfer factor measures gas transfer by assessing carbon monoxide uptake.
    E Peak flows in flow volume loops are MOST affected at high volumes in distal obstruction.

47. Contraindications to surgery for lung carcinoma include all of the following EXCEPT

    A phrenic nerve involvement
    B superior vena cava obstruction
    C oat cell carcinoma
    D FEV_1 1.8 L
    E recurrent laryngeal nerve palsy

48. A 60-year-old dairy farmer presents with fever, cough and shortness of breath. Coarse end-inspiratory crackles are present. Chest x-ray shows bilateral fluffy nodular shadows. The MOST appropriate treatment is

    A amphotericin
    B prednisolone
    C cyclophosphamide
    D salbutamol
    E ciprofloxacin

49. A 40-year-old long-stay patient in a psychiatric hospital presents with fever, abdominal pain, dry cough and worsening confusion. Blood tests reveal neutrophilia, lymphopaenia and hyponatraemia. Chest x-ray shows right-sided lobar consolidation. The MOST appropriate treatment would be

    A erythromycin
    B benzylpenicillin
    C antituberculous chemotherapy
    D ciprofloxacin
    E ticarcillin

50. A 70-year-old man presents with chronic cough, haemoptysis and weight loss. He smokes 20 cigarettes a day. His chest x-ray shows a central coin lesion. The MOST useful investigation would be

    A sputum for culture and cytology
    B isotope bone scan
    C bronchoscopy and biopsy
    D percutaneous needle biopsy
    E chest CT scan

51. A 70-year-old man presents with progressive stepwise dementia associated with focal neurological events. He has a stiff, slow-moving, spastic tongue, dysarthria and inappropriate laughing and crying. He walks with a shuffling gait taking small steps. He is also noted to be hypertensive. The MOST likely diagnosis is

    A Parkinson's disease
    B Alzheimer's disease
    C multi-infarct dementia
    D variant CJD (BSE related)
    E multiple sclerosis

52. The following are types of viral haemorrhagic fever EXCEPT

    A yellow fever
    B Lassa fever
    C Dengue fever
    D Ebola virus
    E relapsing fever

53. Injury to the upper trunk of the brachial plexus affects the following muscles EXCEPT

    A deltoid
    B serratus anterior
    C brachioradialis
    D triceps
    E infraspinatus

54. Charcot's joints are a recognised feature of all the following conditions EXCEPT

    A leprosy
    B diabetes mellitus
    C syringomyelia
    D syphilis
    E rheumatoid arthritis

55. Which ONE of the following features would favour a diagnosis of Guillain–Barré syndrome rather than myasthenia gravis?

    A ocular muscle involvement
    B proximal muscle weakness
    C respiratory difficulties
    D areflexia
    E facial muscle weakness

56. Treatment for multiple sclerosis and its complications includes all of the following EXCEPT

    A glatiramer acetate
    B botulinum toxin
    C interferon beta
    D interferon alfa
    E baclofen

57. The following pairs of neurovascular structures and injuries are correctly paired EXCEPT

   A tibial nerve – proximal fibula fracture
   B sciatic nerve – posterior dislocation of the hip
   C median nerve – Smith's wrist fracture
   D axillary nerve – fracture to humeral neck
   E brachial artery – supracondylar fracture of the humerus

58. Radial nerve injury is associated with all of the following EXCEPT

   A wrist drop
   B weakness of the brachioradialis muscle
   C loss of supinator reflex
   D inability to abduct thumb to 90° to palm
   E wasting of abductor pollicis brevis

59. A 20-year-old man presents with pain on eye movement and double vision after being punched in the eye. On examination he has limitation of upward gaze and anaesthesia over the lateral face and nose. The following injuries are possible EXCEPT

   A blowout fracture
   B inferior rectus entrapment
   C infraorbital nerve injury
   D retinal detachment
   E increased intraorbital pressure

60. The cause of gradual bilateral loss of vision is LEAST likely to be

   A cataract
   B optic atrophy
   C diabetic retinopathy
   D chronic glaucoma
   E choroiditis

61. Eye signs associated with Grave's disease include all of the following EXCEPT

   A exophthalmos
   B proptosis
   C external ophthalmoplegia
   D supraorbital and infraorbital swelling
   E ptosis

62. Recognised treatment for mania include all of the following EXCEPT

    A phenelzine
    B chlorpromazine
    C carbamazepine
    D haloperidol
    E lithium

63. The following are symptoms of schizophrenia EXCEPT

    A obsessional intrusive thoughts
    B thought insertion
    C poverty of speech
    D suspiciousness
    E primary delusion

64. Psychiatric symptoms occur in all of the following physical diseases EXCEPT

    A puerperal infection
    B leprosy
    C nicotinic acid deficiency
    D pernicious anaemia
    E normal pressure hydrocephalus

65. A 20-year-old woman presents with arthralgia and acute jaundice. Markers for hepatitis B infection at this stage include all of the following EXCEPT

    A HBeAg
    B HBsAg
    C IgM anti-HBc
    D Anti-HBe
    E Anti-HBs

66. Coeliac disease is associated with all of the following EXCEPT

    A Vitamin B_{12} deficiency
    B HLA DR3
    C dermatitis herpetiformis
    D steatorrhoea
    E lymphoma

67. Crohn's disease is commonly associated with all of the following EXCEPT

   A gallstones
   B acute ileitis
   C sclerosing cholangitis
   D aphthous ulceration
   E hyperoxaluria

68. The following statements regarding the management of hepatocellular carcinoma (HCC) are correct EXCEPT

   A Partial hepatectomy is the mainstay therapy for early HCC.
   B Hepatitis B infection is a contraindication to liver transplantation.
   C Percutaneous ethanol injection is the MOST commonly used form of local ablative therapy.
   D Transarterial embolisation is relatively contraindicated if the portal system is blocked by tumour invasion.
   E HCC is relatively resistant to systemic chemotherapy.

69. Which ONE of the following features would favour a diagnosis of ulcerative colitis rather than Crohn's disease?

   A uveitis
   B arthritis
   C pyoderma gangrenosum
   D cholelithiasis
   E pseudopolyps

70. Peptic ulcer disease is associated with all of the following EXCEPT

   A head trauma
   B burns
   C chronic pancreatitis
   D hypocalcaemia
   E Helicobacter antral gastritis

71. The following statements regarding bile acids are correct EXCEPT

   A They are absorbed in the ileum.
   B They combine with glycine and taurine to form bile salts.
   C In the intestine they emulsify fats.
   D Cholic acid is a secondary bile acid.
   E Cholesterol is a precursor of the bile acids.

72. The following are causes of megacolon EXCEPT

    A poliomyelitis
    B Crohn's disease
    C Chagas' disease
    D laxative abuse
    E systemic sclerosis

73. The following statements regarding juvenile colonic polyps are correct EXCEPT

    A They are pre-malignant.
    B MOST disappear prior to adulthood.
    C They are rarely symptomatic.
    D They are usually in the sigmoid colon.
    E They may be complicated by rectal prolapse.

74. A 50-year-old woman presents with watery diarrhoea and right iliac fossa pain. On examination a rumbling mid-diastolic murmur is auscultated at the lower left sternal border, louder on inspiration, and the liver is enlarged. 12-lead ECG shows peaked, tall P waves in lead II. The MOST likely diagnosis is

    A VIPoma
    B phaeochromocytoma
    C gastrinoma
    D carcinoid syndrome
    E MEN type I syndrome

75. Sites of carcinoid tumours include all of the following EXCEPT

    A appendix
    B terminal ileum
    C bronchus
    D oesophagus
    E rectum

76. The MOST common cause of significant upper gastrointestinal bleeding is

    A gastric ulcer
    B duodenal ulcer
    C oesophageal varices
    D Mallory–Weiss syndrome
    E angiodysplasia

77. Recognised causes of massive splenomegaly include all of the following EXCEPT

   A malaria
   B bilharzia
   C idiopathic thrombocytopaenic purpura
   D myelofibrosis
   E chronic myeloid leukaemia

78. Risk factors associated with hepatocellular carcinoma include all of the following EXCEPT

   A smoking
   B Clonorchis sinensis
   C vinyl chloride
   D aflatoxins
   E hepatitis B

79. The following statements regarding vitamin D are correct EXCEPT

   A 1,25 (OH)₂ D3 is the MOST active form.
   B 25 (OH) D3 stimulates both calcium and phosphorus absorption in the intestine and the resorption of calcium from bone.
   C Cholecalciferol is synthesised in the skin through the actions of sunlight on 7-dehydrochloesterol.
   D The production of 1,25 (OH)₂ D3 is regulated by parathyroid hormone.
   E The measurement of 25(OH) D3 is a good indicator of vitamin D bioavailability.

80. A 55-year-old insulin-dependent diabetic presents with nausea, lethargy, dry and itchy yellow-brown skin. He also complains of nocturia and impotence. His blood film shows normocytic normochromic anaemia and occasional burr cells. The MOST appropriate management would be

   A Commence iron replacement therapy.
   B Take blood for urea and electrolytes.
   C Check HbA1C.
   D Take blood for bilirubin, LFT's and amylase.
   E Take blood for thyroid function tests.

81. A 20-year-old female presents with acne and hirsutism. She complains of a year of chaotic menstrual cycles with long periods of amenorrhoea. She has gained weight recently. She has never been pregnant. On examination there are no other abnormalities. The MOST likely diagnosis is

A congenital adrenal hyperplasia
B ovarian teratoma
C Cushing's disease
D testicular feminisation
E polycystic ovarian syndrome

82. The type of thyroid carcinoma with the HIGHEST 10-year survival rate is

A follicular
B anaplastic
C medullary
D squamous
E papillary

83. A 50-year-old man presents with polydipsia, headache and weakness. On examination his BP is 160/100 but he is not oedematous. He takes no medication. His blood results reveal hypokalaemia, alkalosis and low serum renin. The MOST likely diagnosis is

A Conn's syndrome
B secondary hyperaldosteronism
C Cushing's disease
D phaeochromocytoma
E renal artery stenosis

84. The following statements regarding gastrin are correct EXCEPT

A It stimulates parietal cells to secrete HCL acid.
B Secretin inhibits gastrin release.
C Somatostatin enhances the release of gastrin.
D It is secreted by G cells in the antrum.
E Duodenal distension enhances the release of gastrin.

85. Functions of cholecystokinin include all of the following EXCEPT

A gallbladder contraction
B pancreatic enzyme secretion
C contraction of the sphincter of Oddi
D inhibition of gastric emptying
E jejunal mucosal enzyme secretion (succus entericus)

86. A patient presents with polydipsia and polyuria, up to 10 L/day. His first morning urine osmolality is 300 mosm/kg. His plasma osmolality is high. He undergoes a water deprivation test. The plasma osmolality rises but the urine osmolality remains dilute. Following desmopressin, the urine osmolality rises to 450 mosm/kg. The MOST likely diagnosis is

A nephrogenic diabetes insipidus
B psychogenic diabetes insipidus
C cranial diabetes insipidus
D SIADH
E diabetes mellitus

87. The following statements regarding vasopressin are correct EXCEPT

A It is synthesised in the posterior pituitary gland.
B It increases peristalsis.
C It increases resorption of water from the distal renal tubules.
D It causes coronary artery vasoconstriction.
E It causes splanchnic bed vasodilatation.

88. Precocious puberty may be associated with all of the following EXCEPT

A hepatoma
B adrenal tumour
C McCune–Albright's syndrome
D Klinefelter's syndrome
E ovarian tumour

89. The following results

Increased serum calcium
Increased serum phosphate
Decreased parathyroid hormone (PTH)
Increased urinary calcium
Increased urinary phosphate

are compatible with which ONE diagnosis?

A vitamin D toxicity
B carcinomatosis
C primary hyperparathyroidism
D secondary hyperparathyroidism
E milk alkali syndrome

90. Diseases associated with impotence include all of the following EXCEPT

   A hyperthyroidism
   B hyperprolactinaemia
   C cirrhosis
   D multiple sclerosis
   E renal failure

91. The following statements regarding thyroid hormones are correct EXCEPT

   A In blood, thyroxine and triiodothyronine are almost entirely bound to plasma proteins.
   B Thyroid stimulating hormone (TSH) stimulates the TSH receptor in the thyroid to release stored hormone.
   C 0.03% of T4 is free hormone.
   D The metabolic state correlates with the total amount of hormone in plasma.
   E 30% of T4 is converted to T3.

92. A 30-year-old dark-tanned man presents with progressive weakness, anorexia, diarrhoea and weight loss. He has just returned from holiday in Cyprus. On examination: BP 100/60. He is noted to have mucosal bluish-black plaques. Blood results

Serum sodium	130 mmol/L
Serum potassium	5 mmol/L
Serum calcium	3 mmol/L
Serum creatinine	200 µmol/L
Serum urea	8 mmol/L

   The MOST likely diagnosis is

   A Addison's disease
   B primary hyperparathyroidism
   C SIADH
   D thyrotoxicosis
   E heavy metal poisoning

93. Characteristic features of distal renal tubular acidosis include all of the following EXCEPT

   A hypokalaemia
   B inability to acidify the urine below pH 5.5
   C hypercalciuria
   D nephrolithiasis
   E association with Fanconi syndrome

94. The MOST common cause of painless frank haematuria in male patients over 50 years old is

   A bladder squamous cell carcinoma
   B carcinoma of the prostate
   C hypernephroma
   D transitional cell carcinoma in the kidney
   E transitional cell bladder carcinoma

95. A 30-year-old man presents to Casualty with a tender swollen testicle. He states that he was struck in the groin while playing football. On examination the border of the testicle is irregular, and the testicle is heavy and woody. There is no associated lymphadenopathy. He is also noted to have gynaecomastia. There are no external signs of trauma. The MOST appropriate initial management would be

   A take blood for α fetoprotein and β-HCG and arrange for a chest x-ray
   B prescribe doxycycline 100 mg o bd × 5 days
   C refer to urologists for urgent surgical exploration
   D arrange for a chest and abdominal CT scan
   E arrange for an ultrasound of the testes

96. The following statements regarding renal tubular disease are correct EXCEPT

   A Hypophosphataemic rickets is due to distal renal tubular unresponsiveness to vitamin D.
   B Cystinosis is associated with proximal renal tubular acidosis (RTA).
   C Osteomalacia is associated with distal RTA.
   D Type I or distal RTA occurs when the tubules fail to create an acid urine.
   E Renal transplantation is associated with proximal RTA.

97. Alport's syndrome is associated with all of the following EXCEPT

   A autosomal dominant inheritance
   B high-frequency sensorineural hearing loss
   C cataract formation
   D bone pain
   E renal tubular disease

98. Cutaneous manifestations of internal malignancy include all the following EXCEPT

   A acquired ichthyosis
   B dermatomyositis
   C thrombophlebitis migrans
   D mycosis fungoides
   E vitiligo

99. Systemic effects of a major burn include all of the following EXCEPT

   A decrease in pulmonary vascular resistance
   B decrease in cardiac output in early burn
   C red cell destruction
   D duodenal mucosa ulceration
   E extravascular fluid and protein loss

100. Type I (von Recklinghausen's) neurofibromatosis is associated with all of the following EXCEPT

   A autosomal dominant inheritance
   B café-au-lait spots
   C acoustic neuromas
   D honeycomb lung
   E axillary freckling

Criterion Referencing Marks

* – 25–50% of candidates expected to get correct
** – 50–75% of candidates expected to get correct
*** – 75–100% of candidates expected to get correct

The notional PASS MARK is 77%

1. A ** The tetrad of Sabin is associated with congenital toxoplasmosis (internal hydrocephalus or microcephaly, chorioretinitis, convulsions and cerebral calcification).

2. B ***

3. C **

4. B *** Shock is associated with increased FFAs.

5. B **

6. D *** Rose spots blanch under pressure.

7. B **

8. E ***

9. B *** Staphylococcus aureus is the organism responsible for toxic shock syndrome.

10. D *** Haemolytic anaemia is associated with a positive direct Coombs' test.

11. D **

12. B ***

13. C ***

14. C ***

15. A *** Haemoglobin consists of 4 globin subunits containing a single haem molecule.

16. D ** The most common cause of death in transplants is from infection.

17. A ***

18. A * Tacrolimus is a calcineurin inhibitor.

19. A ** It is associated with destruction of transfused blood cells by IgG antibodies.

20. E *

21. A ** Octreotide is a somatostatin analogue.

22. B **

23. A *** Tetracycline is a bacteriostatic antibiotic.

24. A ***

25. E **

26. B ***

27. D ** Amantadine is also used to treat Parkinsonism.

28. C **

29. B **

30. E **

31. B ** HLA-B14 and HLA-A3 are associated with idiopathic haemochromatosis.

32. E ** Still's disease is the most common form of juvenile chronic arthritis.

33. C ** Allopurinol is a competitive xanthine oxidase inhibitor.

34. D ***

35. B ***

36. E ***

37. B ***

38. B *** The palmar macules described are Janeway lesions.

39. D *** Verapamil may be used in the presence of β-blockers but with caution to avoid refractory hypotension.

40. D ** Pulsus parvus et tardus is associated with aortic stenosis.

41. B ***

42. A ***

43. D ** Bilharzia is associated with a Type IV hypersensitivity reaction.

44. C * Montelukast may be used in mild to moderate asthma.

45. D *** Cystic fibrosis is associated with chronic infection with pseudomonas aeruginosa.

46. E *** Peak flows in flow volume loops are most affected at low volumes in distal obstruction such as asthma.

47. D ***

48. B ***

49. A ** Erythromycin is the recommended antibiotic for Legionella.

50. C ***

51. C **

52. E **

53. D **

54. E ***

55. D **

56. D ** Glatiramer is a recently introduced immunomodulator.

57. A *** The common peroneal nerve is at risk with a fracture to the proximal neck of the fibular and manifests as a foot drop.

58. E *** Wasting of the abductor pollicis brevis is a sign of median nerve injury.

59. D ***

60. E ** Choroiditis is associated with unilateral loss of vision.

61. E ***

62. A ***

63. A ***

64. B ***

65. E ***

66. A ** Coeliac disease is associated with folate and iron deficiencies even though some malabsorption of B_{12} may occur in the rarely involved terminal ileum it does not lead to deficiency of it.

67. C **

68. B * Hepatitis B is no longer a contraindication to liver transplantation with the advent of antiviral drugs such as lamivudine.

69. E ***

70. D *** Peptic ulcer disease is associated with hypercalcaemia not hypocalcaemia.

71. D *** Bile acids are synthesised and secreted by the liver into bile and converted to secondary bile acids in the small intestine (deoxycholic and lithocolic).

72. B ***

73. A ** Juvenile colonic polyps have no malignancy potential.

74. D ***

75. D ***

76. B ***

77. C ***

78. A ***

79. B *** 1,25 (OH)$_2$ D3 stimulates both calicum and phosphorus absorption in the intestine and the resorption of calcium from bone.

80. B *** This patient has uraemia.

81. E ***

82. E ***

83. A ***

84. C ***

85. C *** CCK relaxes the sphincter of Oddi.

86. C ***

87. A *** Vasopressin is made in the hypothalamus and secreted by the posterior pituitary gland.

88. D **

89. A **

90. A *** Hypothyroidism and not hyperthyroidism is associated with impotence.

91. D ***

92. A ***

93. E *** Fanconi syndrome is associated with proximal RTA.

94. E ***

95. A ***

96. A ** Hypophosphataemic rickets is due to proximal tubular unresponsiveness to vitamin D.

97. D **

98. E ***

99. A ** Major burns are associated with increased pulmonary vascular resistance and Curling's peptic ulcer.

100. C ***

MRCP Paper Five MCQs

Questions

1. Damage to the lowest root of the brachial plexus may result in

   A ptosis
   B clawing of the hand
   C loss of biceps tendon reflex
   D the arm hanging at the side with the forearm pronated and the wrist flexed
   E loss of function of the lumbricals and the interosseous muscles of the hand

2. The median nerve

   A innervates the thenar muscles except adductor pollicis
   B can be tested by opposition of the thumb
   C supplies sensation over the dorsal aspect of the root of the thumb
   D supplies sensation over the entire distal surface of the 4th digit of the hand
   E innervates all the muscles of the thumb except abductor pollicus brevis

3. Hemisection of the spinal cord (Brown–Sequard syndrome) in the upper thoracic region is associated with

   A contralateral spastic paralysis of the leg
   B spinal shock
   C impairment of ipsilateral proprioception below the lesion
   D contralateral analgaesia below the lesion
   E loss of the superficial abdominal reflexes

4. Insulin

   A is a steroid hormone
   B increases glycogenolysis
   C increases amino acid uptake into cells
   D is inhibited by somatostatin
   E is secreted by alpha islet cells

5. Alkaline phosphatase is characteristically raised in the following conditions

   A haemolytic jaundice
   B osteoporosis
   C chronic renal failure
   D multiple myeloma
   E hypoparathyroidism

6. Apoptosis

   A can be seen in viral hepatitis
   B is reversible
   C can be identified histologically
   D occurs in menstruation
   E occurs in myocardial infarction

7. Dystrophic calcification is associated with

   A tuberculosis
   B atheroma
   C hyperparathyroidism
   D ovarian cystadenocarcinoma
   E Monckeberg's sclerosis

8. In a Type I hypersensitivity reaction, mast cells release the following mediators

   A prostaglandin D_2
   B heparin
   C lymphokines
   D bradykinin
   E serotonin

9. The following statements are true

   A The normal (Gaussian) distribution is a bell-shaped, symmetrical curve.
   B The range will give an underestimation of the amount of dispersion if there are extreme scores in a distribution.
   C The mean deviation is derived by subtracting the mean of a distribution from every score in that distribution.
   D The standard deviation is calculated by taking the square root of the variance.
   E The variance is the average of the sum of mean deviations.

10. The following statements are correct

    A The Student's t-test is a parametric test and is used to determine whether differences between groups are significant, when working with categorical rather than score data
    B The chi-square test would be used to compare the blood pressure prior to and following administration of a particular drug
    C Parametric tests are appropriate if the type of data are scores, the value of the scores are normally distributed and the variance of the scores is equal among the group.
    D Non-parametric tests are distribution- free tests
    E The null hypothesis implies a lack of difference between samples and population data

11. Disease manifestations attributable to infection with HIV include

    A Hodgkin's lymphoma
    B disseminated histoplasmosis
    C isospora
    D cerebral toxoplasmosis
    E staphylococcus saprophyticus

12. Coxsackie A virus is associated with

    A herpangina
    B Bornholm disease
    C valvulitis
    D hand, foot, and mouth disease
    E myocarditis

13. Papillary carcinoma of the thyroid

    A is a fast-growing tumour
    B has metastasised to cervical lymph nodes at the time of presentation in about half of patients
    C is encapsulated
    D is associated with increased calcitonin levels
    E represents 70% of thyroid carcinomas

14. Conditions associated with macrocytosis without megaloblastic changes include

    A hyperthyroidism
    B aplastic anaemia
    C alcoholism
    D post-total gastrectomy
    E pernicious anaemia

15. Sickle cell disease (Hb SS) is associated with

    A gallstones
    B renal papillary necrosis
    C priapism
    D Staphylococcal osteomyelitis
    E splenic infarcts

16. The following statements regarding folate are true

    A Folate is destroyed by cooking.
    B Folate deficiency results in microcytosis without megaloblastic change in the bone marrow.
    C Folate deficiency causes peripheral neuropathy.
    D Folate deficiency is associated with phenytoin therapy.
    E Folate deficiency is associated with koilonychia.

17. Causes of haemolytic anaemia include

    A hereditary spherocytosis
    B prosthetic aortic valve
    C mefenamic acid
    D polyarteritis nodosa
    E Haemophilia A

18. Recognised features of Haemophilia B (Christmas disease) include

    A autosomal recessive inheritance
    B abnormal prothrombin time
    C normal bleeding time
    D haemarthroses
    E diagnosis antenatally by chorionic villous biopsy

19. Recognised side-effects of imipramine include

    A sweating
    B increased salivation
    C diarrhoea
    D urinary incontinence
    E hypernatraemia

20. Patients on monoamine-oxidase inhibitors should avoid

    A levodopa
    B aspirin
    C imipramine
    D cheese
    E fluoxetine

21. Drugs associated with inhibition of hepatic enzymes include

A sodium valproate
B phenytoin
C chloramphenicol
D diazepam
E ciprofloxacin

22. Photosensitivity drug eruptions are associated with

A bendrofluazide
B doxycycline
C chlorpropamide
D digoxin
E fluoxetine

23. Increased sensitivity to digoxin is associated with

A concomitant diuretics
B impaired hepatic function
C old age
D recent major surgery
E thyroid disease

24. Constrictive pericarditis

A is most commonly due to a viral infection
B is characterised by ascites and marked peripheral oedema
C may be associated with atrial fibrillation
D may be associated with pulsus alternans
E is associated with a loud high-pitched S1.

25. The following conditions increase cardiac output

A dobutamine
B AV fistula
C Gram-negative septicaemia
D tension pneumothorax
E open chest wound

26. Signs of hypertrophic obstructive cardiomyopathy (HOCM) include

A early systolic aortic ejection murmur
B double impulse at apex
C parasternal heave
D fourth heart sound
E jerky carotid pulse

27. Clinical features of fat embolism include

  A hemiplegia
  B upper thorax petechiae
  C fat globules in retinal blood vessels
  D increased urinary lipases
  E chest pain

28. Haemoptysis is a characteristic feature of

  A tuberculosis
  B Goodpasture's syndrome
  C diffuse interstitial fibrosis
  D pulmonary oedema
  E acute bronchitis

29. Risk factors for pulmonary thromboembolism include

  A recent myocardial infarction
  B progestogen-only pill
  C pelvic fracture
  D alcoholic cirrhosis
  E levonorgestrel intrauterine system contraceptive (Mirena)

30. Acute "Farmers' lung" is associated with

  A Type III immune complex reaction
  B Micropolyspora faeni spores
  C cryptogenic fibrosing alveolitis
  D eosinophilia
  E obstructive changes on spirometry

31. The following statements are true

  A Lung compliance increases with pneumothorax.
  B Lung compliance increases in pulmonary fibrosis.
  C In a normal lung V/Q ratio increases from apex to base.
  D The compliance of the chest wall is defined as change in pulmonary volume divided by unit change in air pressure.
  E Lung compliance decreases in emphysema.

32. Central scotoma is found in

  A posterior occipital lobe lesion
  B multiple sclerosis
  C alcohol optic neuropathy
  D giant-cell arteritis
  E vitamin B_1 deficiency

33. Acoustic neuroma

   A is commonly bilateral
   B may present with sudden deafness
   C presents most often between the ages of 20 and 40
   D may be associated with neurofibromatosis 2
   E represents the majority of cerebellopontine angle tumours

34. Clinical features of vertebro-basilar insufficiency include

   A drop attacks
   B amaurosis fugax
   C ataxia
   D diplopia
   E aphasia

35. In Huntington's disease

   A the EEG shows loss of or reduced β-rhythms
   B the child of an affected parent has a 50% chance of becoming
      affected
   C chorea is treated with dopamine agonists
   D the onset is between 40 and 50 years
   E dementia is an associated feature

36. Adverse side-effects of selective serotonin re-uptake inhibitors include

   A dyskinesias
   B constipation
   C suicidal ideation
   D anxiety associated with abrupt withdrawal
   E delusions

37. Mental changes are seen in

   A fragile × syndrome
   B homocystinuria
   C myxoedema
   D scurvy
   E tuberous sclerosis

38. Bile salts

   A are converted to secondary bile salts in the small intestine
   B increase gut motility
   C are reabsorbed in the colon
   D stimulates bile secretion
   E have a greater detergent action when conjugated with taurine than
      glycine

39. Chronic liver disease is associated with

    A secondary hyperaldosteronism
    B hyperalbuminaemia
    C hypersplenism
    D osteomalacia
    E vitamin B_{12} malabsorption

40. Recognised features of Toxoplasmosis gondii infection include

    A mental retardation
    B cerebral calcification
    C hydrocephalus
    D reactivation by HIV
    E asymptomatic lymphadenopathy

41. The following are used as criteria to determine the severity and prognosis in an attack of acute pancreatitis

    A age
    B serum albumin
    C serum amylase
    D blood neutrophil count
    E arterial oxygen

42. Irritable bowel syndrome is associated with

    A abdominal bloating
    B loss of appetite
    C bleeding per rectum
    D stress
    E food allergy

43. Gastro-oesophageal reflux disease is associated with

    A vagal overactivity
    B rapid gastric emptying
    C Barrett's oesophagus
    D H. pylori infection
    E odynophagia

44. The following statements regarding human immunodeficiency virus (HIV) are correct

   A A patient with a viral load of >30,000 and a CD4 count of <200 has an 85% risk of developing AIDS within 3 years.
   B Anti-HIV treatment should be started when the viral load is in the 10,000 to 20,000 range, even if the CD4 count is high.
   C Regular viral load tests are recommended every 6 months when on treatment.
   D Drug resistance does not develop at viral load levels between 50 and 500.
   E Risk of pneumocystis carinii pneumonia occurs at a CD4 count of 300.

45. Osteomalacia is associated with

   A fractures of the femoral shaft
   B bone pain
   C proximal myopathy
   D decreased alkaline phosphatase
   E increased serum phosphate

46. In osteoporosis in women

   A oestrogen increases bone mass
   B raloxifene is a recognised treatment
   C a decrease in the number and size of the trabecullae in woven bone is characteristic
   D hormone replacement therapy (HRT) should be discontinued 6 weeks before major elective surgery
   E bisphosphonates decrease the risk of vertebral fractures in post-menopausal women

47. Evidence-based medicine

   A is restricted to randomised trials and meta-analyses
   B suggests that the standard for judging the efficacy of a treatment should be based on the systematic review of several randomised trials
   C suggests we determine the accuracy of a diagnostic test by a randomised trial of patients harbouring the relevant disorder
   D is an attempt to lower the cost of patient's care
   E involves using the best available external evidence to treat a patient

48. The following statements regarding thyroid cancer are true

A Prior to surgery in medullary carcinoma patients should be screened for phaeochromocytoma.
B The commonest carcinoma is papillary.
C Follicular carcinoma tends to occur in patients under 30 years of age.
D Follicular carcinoma cannot be diagnosed on fine-needle aspirate cytology.
E Hyperthyroidism commonly occurs in well differentiated follicular carcinoma.

49. Type I insulin-dependent diabetes mellitus is associated with

A a 100% concordance in identical twins
B islet cell antibodies at the time of diagnosis
C HLA-DR2
D Class I major histocompatibility complexes
E a more frequent presentation in the summer

50. Haematuria is a characteristic feature of

A hydronephrosis
B renal cell carcinoma
C porphyria
D adult polycystic kidney disease
E rifampicin administration

51. Retroperitoneal fibrosis is associated with

A dilation and lateral deviation of the ureters
B increased incidence in women
C abdominal aortic aneurysm
D stomach carcinoma
E IgG-mediated periaortitis

52. Causes of nephrotic syndrome include

A sickle cell disease
B malaria
C IgA nephropathy (Berger's disease)
D focal segmental glomerulosclerosis
E rapidly progressive glomerulonephritis

53. Regarding renal involvement in systemic lupus erythematosus

   A prognosis is worse with membranous lesions than with proliferative GN
   B cyclophosphamide improves renal function
   C nephrotic syndrome may occur
   D corticosteroids have no effect on renal prognosis
   E it is associated with anti-GBM antibodies

54. Adult polycystic disease of the kidney is associated with

   A cysts in the liver in 30% of cases
   B a single gene defect linked to the α-haemoglobin gene locus on the short arm of chromosome 6
   C hepatic failure
   D polycythaemia
   E subarachnoid haemorrhage

55. Acute nephritic syndrome may be a complication of

   A Lancefield group A beta-haemolytic streptococcus infection
   B systemic lupus erythematosus
   C polyarteritis nodosa
   D amyloidosis
   E Wegener's granulomatosis

56. Sjogren's syndrome

   A always affects the salivary glands
   B is characterised by periductal lymphocytes in multiple organs
   C is associated with primary biliary cirrhosis
   D may progress to carcinoma of the tongue
   E is associated with crocodile tears – lacrimation during eating

57. Avascular necrosis is associated with

   A supracondylar fracture of the femur
   B fracture of the talus
   C fracture of the scaphoid
   D posterior dislocation of the hip
   E posterior dislocation of the shoulder

58. Hirsutism is associated with

   A adrenogenital syndrome
   B polycystic ovarian disease
   C minoxidil
   D cimetidine
   E hyperthyroidism

59. Malignant melanoma

  A has a worse prognosis if it arises in the BANS region (back, back of arms, neck or scalp).
  B when of lentigo melanoma type is the most aggressive
  C rarely appears on the palms or soles
  D rarely arises in the black population
  E responds to treatment with IL-2

60. Otosclerosis

  A is a hereditary disease which can skip generations
  B involves the stapes
  C is rarely bilateral
  D improves with each pregnancy
  E tinnitus in most cases

Answers to Paper Five MCQs

Criterion Referencing Marks

    *   – 25–50% of candidates expected to get correct
    **   – 50–75% of candidates expected to get correct
    *** – 75–100% of candidates expected to get correct

The notional PASS MARK is 204/300 or 68%

1. TTFFT ** C8/T1 lesions may be associated with Horner's syndrome or Klumpke's palsy. The fourth option describes Erb–Duchenne's palsy of C5/C6.

2. TTFFF *** The radial nerve innervates sensation at the dorsal root of the thumb. Sensation over the distal tip of the ring finger is shared with the ulnar nerve.

3. FTTTF ** Brown-Sequard syndrome is characterised by ipsilateral spastic paralysis and contralateral analgaesia due to crossing of spinothalamic tract.

4. FFTTF *** Insulin is a peptide and is secreted by the β-cells.

5. FFTFF ***

6. TFTTF ** Apoptosis is defined as genetically programmed cell death and is part of normal development. It involves macrophages and requires an intact cell membrane.

7. TTFTT * Hyperparathyroidism is an example of metastatic calcification.

8. TTFTT * Other mediators released by mast cells include histamine, SRS-A and platelet-activating factor.

9. TFTTF ** The range would be overestimated in this situation. The variance is the average of the sum of square deviations.

10. FFTTT* The definitions for Student t-test and chi-square are reversed. Parametric tests include Student t-tests and chi-square.

11. FTTTF *** Non-Hodgkins lymphoma occurs in AIDS patients. Staphylococcus saprophyticus causes UTIs in young women and has no relation to AIDS. Other opportunistic infections include CMV, mycobacterium avium intracellulare, bronchial or pulmonary candidiasis and pneumocystis carinii pneumonia.

12. TFFTF ** Coxsackie B and not A virus is associated with Bornholm disease (intercostal muscle involvement, lymphocytic meningitis, and myocarditis). Valvulitis is also associated with Coxsackie B virus.

13. FTFFT **

14. TTTFF ** Other macrocytic anaemias with normoblastic bone marrow include pregnancy, hepatic cirrhosis, sideroblastic anaemia, hypothyroidism, and reticulocytosis.

15. TTTFT *** Sickle cell disease is associated with Salmonella osteomyelitis and bacterial septicaemia. Sickle cell trait (Hb AS) is associated with polyuria and also affords protection against Plasmodium falciparum malaria.

16. TFFTF ** Folate deficiency results in a megaloblastic anaemia. Dietary folate deficiency accounts for 1/5th of the causes of megaloblastic anaemia in the UK. Severe folate deficiency is associated with glossitis and hypersegmented neutrophils. Treatment of Vitamin B_{12} deficiency by folate may cause peripheral neuropathy.

17. TTTFF *** Other causes of haemolytic anaemia include hereditary elliptocytosis, accelerated hypertension, and Wilson's disease.

18. FFTTT ** Haemophilia B like A is an X-linked recessive condition. Lack of Factor IX leads to a prolonged APTT.

19. TFFFF ** Side-effects of tricyclic antidepressants include dry mouth, sweating, constipation and urinary retention. Hyponatraemia may occur in the elderly.

20. TTTTT **

21. TFTFT ** Other drugs associated with inhibition of hepatic enzymes include cimetidine, indomethacin, suphonamides and tamoxifen.

22. TTTFF * Drugs associated with photosensitivity reactions include thiazides, amiodarone, terbinafine, tetracyclines, phenothiazines, sulphonamides, NSAIDs, nalidixic acid and chlorpropamide.

23. TFTFT * Increased sensitivity to digoxin is associated with renal impairment and hypokalaemia.

24. FTTFF *** The most common cause of constrictive pericarditis is tuberculous pericarditis. Other causes include acute viral or bacterial pericarditis and haemopericarditis. Constrictive pericarditis is associated with a pulsus paradoxus, right heart failure, and a pericardial knock (loud high-pitched S2 not S1). It is also a post-hepatic cause of portal hypertension. On 50% of chest x-rays, the characteristic small heart with obvious calcifications may be seen.

25. TTTFF *** Tension pneumothorax and an open chest wound are associated with a decrease in cardiac output.

26. FTFTT *** HOCM is associated with a late systolic murmur, a left ventricular tract outflow gradient and may be associated with a pansystolic murmur of mitral regurgitation.

27. TTTTF *

28. TTFFF ***

29. TFTFT ***

30. TTFFF ** Acute farmers' lung is a Type III (immune complex) reaction to Micropolyspora faeni spores. It is a form of extrinsic allergic alveolitis and elicits restrictive changes on RFTs. There is a neutrophilia but the eosinophil count is normal. Expected lung findings include crackles and precipitating antibodies in the blood to thermophilic actinomycetes.

31. FFFTF ** Lung compliance increases with emphysema. In a normal lung the V/Q ratio increases from base to apex.

32. TTTTF ** Central scotomas are blind-spots often associated with optic nerve pathology. Multiple sclerosis gives rise to optic neuritis. Giant-cell arteritis is a form of ischaemic optic neuropathy. Vitamin B_{12} deficiency and not B_1 is associated with optic neuropathy. The posterior pole of the occipital cortex is where central vision is represented; as it lies at the "watershed" of middle and posterior cerebral artery territories macular sparing sometimes occurs with occlusion of the latter.

33. FTFTT **Acoustic neuroma may be bilateral in cases of NF2. It presents more often between the ages of 40 and 60.

34. TFTTF *** Other features of vertebro-basilar insufficiency include vomiting, vertigo, dysarthria, hemisensory loss and hemianopic visual loss.

35. FTFTT ** EEG shows loss of α-rhythms. Treatment of chorea is with dopamine antagonists.

36. TFTTF ** Adverse side-effects of SSRIs include hyponatraemia, GI upset and abrupt withdrawal syndrome (paresthesiae, dizziness, anxiety, nausea, headache).

37. TTTFT ***

38. TTFTF * Bile salts are reabsorbed in the ileum.

39. TFTTF *** Chronic liver disease is associated with hypoalbuminaemia. Osteomalacia results from derangement of vitamin D metabolism.

40. TTTTT ***

41. TTFTT ***

42. TFFTF ***

43. TFTFT ***

44. TTFFF * Regular viral load tests are recommended every 2–3 months when on treatment. Risk of PCP occurs at CD4 counts of <200.

45. FTTFF *** Osteomalacia is associated with fractures of the neck of the femur not the shaft and pseudo fractures (Looser's zones). Calcium and phosphate levels are low and alkaline phosphatase is elevated. Osteomalacia may be associated with secondary hyperparathyroidism.

46. FTFTT ** Oestrogen limits the loss of bone mass. Raloxifene is a selective oestrogen receptor modulator used in treatment. Osteoporosis affects the trabeculae of cancellous bone. One in two women over 70 will develop an osteoporotic-related fracture.

47. FTFFF ** Evidence-based medicine involves using both individual clinical expertise and the best available external evidence to determine patient's care. The accuracy of a diagnostic test should be determined by finding proper cross-sectional studies of patients harbouring the disorder. Evidence-based medicine may raise the cost of patients' care.

48. TTFFF ** Follicular carcinoma usually presents after age 30. Papillary carcinoma presents at age <30 years. Follicular carcinoma cannot be diagnosed at FNAC, as malignancy is determined by capsular invasion; follicular carcinoma is encapsulated; it rarely causes hyperthyroidism.

49. FTFFF ** NIDDM is associated with a 100% concordance in identical twins; for IDDM the figure is 30–50%. HLA-DR2 is associated with a decreased risk of IDDM. 95% of IDDM patients have HLA-DR3, DR4 or both. The class I MHC includes HLA-A, B and C not DR. The class II MHC includes HLA-DR antigens. It is suggested that there is a link between seasonal viral triggers of IDDM, more often during the spring and autumn seasons. 70% of patients have islet cell IgG antibodies at presentation.

50. FTFTF *** Grawitz tumour also known as hypernephroma or renal cell carcinoma is the most common renal tumour in adults.

51. FFTFT ** Retroperitoneal fibrosis is associated with medial deviation of the ureters. It is commonly seen in middle-aged men and may also be associated with abdominal aortic aneurysm, bladder or colon carcinoma or retroperitoneal lymphoma. Hypertension is a recognised complication.

52. TTFTF *** Other causes of nephrotic syndrome include membranous glomerulonephritis (GN), minimal change GN, membranoproliferative GN, captopril, D-penicillamine therapy, SBE, SLE, PAN, DM and amyloid.

53. FTTTF ** Prognosis is better with membranous GN than proliferative GN.

54. TFFTT ** Adult polycystic kidney disease affects chromosome 16 not 6.

55. TTTFT ** Acute nephritic syndrome is most often associated with post-strep infection. Other associations include Henoch–Schönlein purpura, mesangial IgA nephropathy and mesangio-capillary GN.

56. FTTFF ** Sjogren's syndrome affects the salivary glands in 40% of cases. Secondary Sjogren's syndrome is associated with connective tissue disorders. Bell's palsy is associated with crocodile tears. Sjogren's syndrome is characterised by xerostomia or xerophthalmia or both. B cell lymphoma is a recognised complication.

57. FTTTF ***

58. TTTFF **

59. TFFFF ** Malignant melanoma has a worse prognosis if the site involved is the trunk or BANS region. Nodular melanoma has the worst prognosis. Acral lentiginous melanoma appears on the palms, soles or subungual regions and is more common in Asians and blacks. Immunotherapy has not had promising results.

60. TTFFT **

MRCP Paper Five BOFs

In these questions candidates must select one answer only

Questions

1. The following are transmitted by insect vectors EXCEPT

   A Wucheria bancrofti
   B Plasmodia falciparum
   C Leishmania
   D Trypanosoma brucei gambiense
   E Ascariasis

2. Pelvic inflammatory disease is associated with all of the following EXCEPT

   A infertility
   B ectopic pregnancies
   C Chlamydia trachomatis infection
   D tubo-ovarian abscess
   E endometriosis

3. The MOST common viral illness in transplant patients is

   A human immunodeficiency virus
   B herpes zoster
   C herpes simplex
   D cytomegalovirus
   E Epstein–Barr virus

4. A 20-year-old man returned from hitchhiking through South America a fortnight ago now presents with explosive watery foul-smelling diarrhoea and weight loss. On examination he has abdominal distension. His stools are greasy and contain mucus. The MOST useful investigation would be

   A proctoscopy
   B sodium sweat test
   C abdominal x-ray
   D stool for microscopy
   E duodenal aspirate

5. A 25-year-old man presents with a short history of fatigue and myalgia. The differential diagnosis includes all of the following EXCEPT

A cytomegalovirus
B infectious mononucleosis
C chronic fatigue syndrome (ME syndrome)
D toxoplasmosis
E prodromal herpes zoster

6. A 24-year-old African man presents to Casualty with acute onset of fever, vomiting, jaundice and dark brown-black urine. He had been travelling through Africa 6 weeks ago and had taken chloroquine prophylaxis. He is not taking any medication now. On examination he has irregular fever patterns and a BP 100/60. There is hepatosplenomegaly, hypertonia and hyper-reflexia. Serum urea and creatinine are markedly elevated and haemoglobinuria is present. The MOST likely diagnosis is

A Plasmodium malariae
B Plasmodium falciparum
C African trypanosomiasis
D Yellow Fever
E Leishmaniasis

7. A 30-year-old man presents with fever and jaundice. He enjoys travelling and water sports and has recently returned from Sri Lanka. On examination he is also noted to have injected conjunctivae and hepatomegaly. His Hb is low, and he has microscopic haematuria. ESR, serum creatinine and urea are markedly raised, and his serum transaminases are only slightly raised. The MOST likely diagnosis is

A relapsing fever
B leptospira ictero haemorrhagica (Weil's disease)
C yellow fever
D Q fever
E leishmaniasis

8. The treatment of choice is

A metronidazole
B penicillin
C ciprofloxacin
D tetracycline
E doxycycline

9. The following statements regarding Christmas Disease are correct EXCEPT

A It is the second most common congenital coagulopathy.
B It is associated with Factor IX deficiency.
C It may be corrected with cryoprecipitate.
D It may cause severe bleeding post-injury.
E It may be corrected with fresh frozen plasma.

10. Primary tumours associated with bone metastases include all of the following EXCEPT

A kidney
B breast
C prostate
D thyroid
E lung

11. Recognised complications of blood replacement by blood transfusion include all of the following EXCEPT

A hypothermia
B hyperkalaemia
C hypercalcaemia
D metabolic acidosis
E thrombocytopaenia

12. Of the factors in Hodgkin's disease the one which carries the BEST prognosis is

A age greater than 50
B absence of constitutional symptoms
C lymphocyte depletion histologically
D female
E nodular sclerosis histologically

13. Chemical mediators of increased vascular permeability include all of the following EXCEPT

A C3b
B bradykinin
C histamine
D serotonin
E leukotriene

14. Post-splenectomy complications include all of the following EXCEPT

   A falciparum malaria
   B haemophilus influenza infection
   C pneumococcal septicaemia
   D thrombo-embolism
   E thrombocytopaenia

15. The following pairs of antibiotics and mechanisms of action have been correctly paired EXCEPT

   A penicillin   inhibits cell wall synthesis
   B clavulanic acid   inhibits β-lactamase
   C erythromycin   inhibits protein synthesis in ribosome
   D gentamicin   inhibits folic acid synthesis
   E trimethoprim   inhibits dihydrofolate reductase

16. The following statements regarding ACE inhibitors are correct EXCEPT

   A ACE inhibitors are recommended within 24 hours of a myocardial infarction in a normotensive patient without any contraindications.
   B They should be avoided in insulin-dependent diabetics with nephropathy.
   C They are indicated for hypertension when thiazides and β-blockers are contraindicated or have been less effective.
   D They should be used cautiously in patients receiving diuretics.
   E They cause severe renal failure in patients with bilateral renal artery stenosis.

17. The following statements regarding β-blockers are correct EXCEPT

   A Carvedilol is recommended for patients with stable heart failure and left-ventricular systolic dysfunction.
   B Atenolol is contraindicated in NIDDM type II diabetes.
   C Sotalol is indicated for prophylaxis of paroxysmal atrial tachycardia.
   D Propranolol is contraindicated in patients with COAD.
   E Sudden withdrawal of propranolol may cause an exacerbation of angina.

18. The following antibiotics and their recognised complications have been correctly paired EXCEPT

   A chloramphenicol – aplastic anaemia
   B neomycin – nephrotoxicity
   C cephalosporin – bleeding dyscrasia
   D penicillin – bone marrow suppression
   E trimethoprim – teeth mottling

19. A 30-year-old man presents in coma following drug overdose. His pupils are dilated, and he is hypotensive. His pulse rate drops to 40 and ECG confirms second degree Mobitz type II heart block. The MOST likely cause of his overdose is

A barbiturate
B tricyclic antidepressant
C lithium
D β-blocker
E benzodiazepine

20. Recognised side-effects of thiazide diuretics include all of the following EXCEPT:

A hyperuricaemia
B increased LDL cholesterol
C hypokalaemia
D hypoglycaemia
E hypercalcaemia

21. The first-line therapy for hypertension in a pregnant woman is

A atenolol
B hydralazine
C methyldopa
D bendrofluazide
E nifedipine

22. The following are recognised treatment for migraine EXCEPT

A methysergide
B calcium channel blocker
C tricyclic antidepressant
D β-blocker
E serotonin antagonist

23. The treatment of choice for adolescent-onset Gilles de la Tourette's syndrome is

A ritalin
B pimozide
C haloperidol
D clonidine
E clonazepam

24. Sodium valproate is associated with all of the following EXCEPT

   A transient alopecia
   B Stevens–Johnson syndrome
   C ataxia
   D gynaecomastia
   E thrombocytosis

25. An 8-year-old recently adopted boy presents with painful swelling of the right knee. On examination there is joint subluxation and an effusion present. There is also wasting of the right quadriceps. Aspiration confirms haemarthrosis. The MOST likely diagnosis is

   A apophysitis of the tibial tubercle (Osgood–Schlatter disease)
   B haemophilia
   C juvenile rheumatoid arthritis
   D non-accidental injury (NAI)
   E Still's disease

26. A 40-year-old woman presents with fever, symmetrical polyarthralgia affecting the fingers, wrists and knees, and weight loss. She is also noted to have alopecia, oral and nasal mucosal ulceration. Her full blood count shows anaemia with thrombocytopaenia. Her ESR is raised. The MOST definitive investigation is

   A rheumatoid factor
   B ANA
   C anticentromere antibodies
   D antibodies to double-stranded DNA
   E c-ANCA

27. A 15-year-old boy presents with high swinging fever and arthritis affecting the knees. The joints are swollen but not very tender. His blood tests reveal anaemia and a raised ESR. Rheumatoid factor is negative but antinuclear antibodies are positive. The MOST likely diagnosis is

   A acute rheumatic fever
   B juvenile rheumatoid arthritis
   C Still's disease
   D osteochondritis dissecans
   E aseptic non-traumatic synovitis

28. The NEXT most appropriate step to guide your further management is

    A echocardiography
    B aspiration of knee joint
    C arrange for MRI scan of the knee
    D arrange for ophthalmology referral for slit-lamp examination
    E blood cultures

29. A 40-year-old man has inadvertently been given adrenaline IV for anaphylactic shock. He is now in supraventricular tachycardia with a rate of 180/min. His blood pressure is 100/60. Oxygen is administered and vagal manoeuvres are attempted without success. The NEXT most appropriate management would be

    A up to three synchronised DC shocks at 100J: 200J: 360J
    B adenosine 6 mg IV bolus
    C verapamil 5–10 mg IV
    D amiodarone 150 mg IV over 10 min
    E amiodarone 300 mg IV over 1 hr

30. Despite your measures, he now complains of chest pain and his rate has increased to 210/min. The most appropriate management NOW would be

    A amiodarone 150 mg IV over 10 min
    B esmolol 40 mg over 1 min followed by infusion at 4 mg/min
    C verapamil 5–10 mg IV
    D digoxin 500 μg IV over 30 min
    E up to three synchronised DC shocks at 100J: 200J: 360J

31. A 60-year-old man collapses on the ward. ECG shows asystole. There is no palpable carotid pulse. The MOST appropriate management is

    A DC cardioversion starting at 200 J
    B 1 min of CPR during which the airway is secured and 1 mg of adrenaline IV is administered
    C 3 mins of CPR during which the airway is secured and 3 mg of atropine IV is administered
    D repeated precordial blows at a rate of 70/min (percussion pacing)
    E 3 mins of CPR during which the airway is secured and both adrenaline and atropine IV are administered

32. A 70-year-old man presents with calf pain upon exercise, which disappears with rest. He smokes 20 cigarettes a day and takes bendrofluazide for hypertension. He has weak posterior tibial and dorsalis pedis pulses. His ankle-brachial Doppler index is 0.7. All of the following should be considered in his immediate management EXCEPT

A arteriogram
B oxypentifylline
C low dose aspirin
D naftidrofuryl
E stop smoking

33. A 70-year-old man presents with nausea, vomiting and weakness. He has marked peripheral oedema. His medications include digoxin and chlorthalidone for congestive heart failure. Frusemide is administered to which he has marked diuresis of 10 litres and promptly collapses. His ECG shows prolonged P-R interval, inverted T waves and depressed ST segments. The MOST likely complication to have occurred is

A transient cardiac arrhythmia
B acute renal failure
C myocardial infarction
D hypoxia
E hypovolaemia

34. A 50-year-old man with a history of previous myocardial infarction presents to Casualty with chest pain. His initial blood pressure is 110/70. During evaluation, he collapses. His ECG shows ventricular tachycardia. He has no palpable pulse. The MOST appropriate management would be

A synchronised DC shock at 100J
B administer IV amiodarone 150 mg over 10 mins
C DC cardioversion with 200J
D administer IV lignocaine 50 mg over 2 mins
E commence CPR

35. A 60-year-old man is brought to casualty unconscious. His BP is 60/40, and his pulse rate is 35/min. ECG shows Mobitz type II AV block. He does not respond to a total of 3 mg IV of atropine. The DEFINITIVE treatment for this patient is

A transcutaneous pacing
B adrenaline infusion titrated to response
C transvenous pacing
D synchronised DC shock
E percussion pacing

36. A 30-year-old woman presents with fever and a sharp, constant sub-sternal chest pain. She is clutching her chest and leaning forward in her chair. ECG shows ST-elevation in leads V2-6 and in the limb leads except aVR. Several days later the T-wave inverts in these same leads. The MOST likely diagnosis at presentation is

A post-myocardial infarction syndrome (Dressler's syndrome)
B pulmonary embolism
C coronary artery spasm (Prinzmetal's angina)
D myocardial infarction
E pericarditis

37. Cystic fibrosis is associated with all of the following EXCEPT

A autosomal recessive inheritance
B absent testes
C raised immunoreactive trypsin in affected babies
D deletion of the codon for phenylalanine at position 508 on the long arm of chromosome 7
E nasal polyps

38. Positive end-expiratory pressure ventilation is associated with all of the following EXCEPT

A increased cardiac output
B pneumothorax
C decreased right-to-left shunt
D increased functional residual capacity
E increased arterial oxygen content

39. Extrapulmonary effects of lung carcinoma include all of the following EXCEPT

A syndrome of inappropriate antidiuretic hormone (SIADH)
B carcinoid syndrome
C hypertrophic pulmonary osteoarthropathy
D thrombangiitis obliterans
E Eaton–Lambert syndrome

40. A 50-year-old man complains of dry cough. He is noted to have facial telangiectasias and finger clubbing. On auscultation he has fine-inspiratory crepitations. Chest x-ray shows increased interstitial markings. Lung function tests reveal reduced lung volumes. Bronchoalveolar lavage shows a predominance of neutrophils. The MOST likely diagnosis is

A cryptogenic fibrosing alveolitis
B mesothelioma
C systemic sclerosis
D sarcoidosis
E miliary tuberculosis

41. A 50-year-old obese man presents with headache and drowsiness. He has a history of snoring. He has warm extremities, a flapping tremor and a bounding pulse. On fundoscopic examination papilloedema is present. The MOST likely cause for the papilloedema is

A CO_2 retention (hypercapnia)
B hypoxia
C obstructive sleep apnoea
D cerebral tumour
E malignant hypertension

42. A 25-year-old woman presents to Casualty with light-headedness and breathlessness. She complains of tingling and numbness of her hands. Arterial blood gas:

pH	7.55
$PaCO_2$	3 kPa
PaO_2	14 kPa
H^+	25 nmol/L
HCO_3	20 mmol/L

The MOST appropriate management would be

A chest x-ray
B breathe into a paper bag
C activated charcoal
D needle thoracentesis
E V/Q scan

43. A 20-year-old asthmatic presents with increased shortness of breath. On chest examination he is found to have a deviated trachea to the right, reduced tactile fremitus and hyperresonance to percussion on the left. The MOST likely diagnosis is

A right-sided pulmonary embolism
B right-sided pneumothorax
C left-sided pneumothorax
D left bronchopneumonia
E left-sided pleural effusion

44. A 12-year-old boy presents to Casualty with severe dyspnoea. He had been treated by his GP with penicillin for presumed tonsillitis. He uses a salbutamol inhaler for asthma. On examination: temperature 40°C and he is drooling saliva; no trismus. Marked inspiratory stridor and a respiratory rate of 30/min. The MOST appropriate management would be

A oxygen-driven nebuliser
B IV hydrocortisone
C indirect laryngoscopy
D endotracheal intubation under general anaesthesia
E cricothyroidotomy

45. The MOST likely diagnosis is

A croup
B acute epiglottitis
C glandular fever
D acute streptococcal tonsillitis
E acute severe asthma attack

46. A 50-year-old man presents with facial cellulitis. It extends from the front of his forehead down over the bridge of his nose. On fundoscopic examination he has papilloedema. Your MAIN concern is

A meningitis
B cavernous sinus thrombosis
C orbital abscess
D trigeminal herpes zoster
E erysipelas

47. A 50-year-old obese man is brought to Casualty in a confused state. On examination he has nystagmus and is unable to move the eyes fully laterally. He walks with a broad-based gait. He is unaware of his surroundings and grows restless. The MOST appropriate management is

A 50 ml of 50% dextrose IV
B parenteral vitamins B and C (pabrinex) IM
C hydroxocobalamin IM
D oral folic acid
E urgent head CT scan

48. A 40-year-old woman presents with painful eyes and blurred vision. On examination she is found to have a relative afferent pupillary defect and internuclear ophthalmoplegia. On fundoscopic exam there is bilateral papilloedema. Bilateral positive Babinski sign is elicited. The MOST likely diagnosis is

A aneursym of posterior communicating artery (of circle of Willis)
B transverse myelitis
C neuromyelitis optica (Devic syndrome)
D SLE
E diabetes mellitus

49. A 30-year-old man presents with a left winged scapula, demonstrated by pushing against a wall with both hands. The nerve that has been affected is

A long thoracic
B dorsal scapular
C suprascapular
D lateral pectoral
E thoracodorsal

50. A 12-year-old girl presents with gradual right hearing loss associated with tinnitus and headache. She denies trauma to the ears and is up-to-date with her immunisations including MMR. The tympanic membrane appears normal. Pure-tone audiogram demonstrates right sensorineural hearing loss. The DEFINITIVE investigation would be

A head CT scan
B MRI of the brain with gadolinium enhancement
C lumbar puncture
D viral titres
E brainstem electric response audiometry

51. The MOST likely diagnosis is

    A herpes zoster oticus (Ramsay–Hunt syndrome)
    B measles virus
    C mumps virus
    D neurofibromatosis type II
    E neurofibromatosis type I

52. A 30-year-old woman presents with bilateral ptosis and diplopia. She has also noticed difficulty in swallowing. The MOST likely diagnosis is

    A dystrophia myotonica
    B multiple sclerosis
    C polymyositis
    D myasthenic syndrome (Eaton–Lambert syndrome)
    E myasthenia gravis

53. A 20-year-old woman presents with complete right ptosis. On lifting the eyelid, the eye is seen to be looking down and out. The pupil is dilated. The MOST likely diagnosis is

    A right third nerve and right fourth nerve palsy
    B complete right third nerve palsy
    C incomplete right third nerve palsy
    D Horner's syndrome
    E right third nerve and sixth nerve palsy

54. The MOST common cause of new-onset focal or generalised seizures after the age of 50 is:

    A alcoholism
    B brain abscess
    C brain tumour
    D cerebrovascular disease
    E encephalitis

55. A 40-year-old woman complains of progressive difficulty climbing and descending stairs, rising from a chair or reaching for an object on a top shelf. This has been going on for several months. She has no ocular symptoms but does have mild difficulty swallowing. There is no family history of neurological disorders. On examination her sensation and reflexes are normal. She has some proximal muscle weakness and atrophy. The MOST likely diagnosis is

A myasthenia gravis
B multiple sclerosis
C polymyositis
D motor neurone disease
E myasthenic syndrome (Eaton–Lambert syndrome)

56. A 30-year-old man presents with a right red painful eye. He complains of watering of the eyes and sensitivity to light. He has a history of recurrent cold sores. Fluorescein staining of the cornea demonstrates a tree-shaped sharp-bordered stain. The MOST likely diagnosis is

A dendritic ulcer
B keratoconjunctivitis sicca
C corneal abrasion
D corneal ulcer
E conjunctivitis

57. A 20-year-old woman presents to Casualty with an excruciatingly painful right red eye. She states that her child accidentally poked her in the eye. Her visual acuity and colour vision are both normal. Fluorescein dye confirms a corneal abrasion. The MOST appropriate management would be

A topical application of local anaesthetic
B double eye padding for 48 hours
C refer urgently to ophthalmologist
D arrange for orbital ultrasound
E hypomellose eye lubricant for 2 months

58. The following conditions can mimic panic disorder EXCEPT

A phaeochromocytoma
B hyperthyroidism
C hypoglycaemia
D caffeine withdrawal
E barbiturate withdrawal

59. A 20-year-old man presents for psychotherapy. He is manipulative and lacks empathy. He has a grandiose sense of self-importance and entitlement. The MOST likely personality disorder would be described as

A antisocial
B borderline
C histrionic
D schizotypal
E narcissistic

60. A 22-year-old female presents with secondary amenorrhoea and weight loss. On examination she is noted to have mild parotid swelling. She has a low BP and a body mass index (BMI) of 15. The MOST likely reason for her amenorrhoea is

A prolactinoma
B Addison's disease
C premature ovarian failure
D anorexia nervosa
E bulimia

61. The following are first-rank symptoms of schizophrenia EXCEPT

A anhedonia
B bodily sensations being imposed by an outside agency
C delusional perceptions
D third person auditory hallucinations
E alien thoughts

62. Risk factors for cholelithiasis include all of the following conditions EXCEPT

A Crohn's disease
B haemolytic diseases
C multiparity
D males greater than 40 years of age
E contraceptive pill

63. A 20-year-old woman presents with a temperature of 40°C and a week of bloody diarrhoea. She looks unwell and dehydrated. She has been taking erythromycin for 3 months for acne. She has not travelled abroad, and no one else in the family is unwell. The MOST appropriate management would be

    A routine stool culture and microscopy
    B admit to hospital, hydrate, take a prompt, direct faecal smear and culture and commence ciprofloxacin
    C refer to consultant GI surgeon's outpatient clinic
    D admit to hospital, hydrate and request measure C. difficile toxin in stool with stool culture and microscopy
    E admit to hospital and request urgent GI surgeon consultation

64. Causes of acalculous cholecystitis include all of the following EXCEPT

    A Lassa fever
    B typhoid fever
    C actinomycosis
    D scarlet fever
    E ascariasis

65. A 50-year-old man presents with weight loss, hiccoughs, jaundice, epigastric and right upper quadrant pain radiating to the back. On examination he is noted to have hepatomegaly, a palpable gallbladder and an abdominal bruit heard in the periumbilical area and left upper quadrant. The MOST likely diagnosis is

    A abdominal aortic aneurysm
    B gallbladder carcinoma
    C hepatocellular carcinoma
    D carcinoma of the head of the pancreas
    E cholecystitis

66. A 43-year-old man complains of epigastric discomfort, griping widespread abdominal pain and frequent bowel action. There is mucus in the stools. Gastroscopy, abdominal ultrasound, sigmoidoscopy, and barium enema are all normal. The MOST appropriate management would be to give reassurance and

    A mebeverine
    B diazepam
    C metoclopropamide
    D omeprazole
    E loperamide

67. A 62-year-old woman who has recently undergone liver transplantation for primary biliary cirrhosis presents with pruritis and right upper quadrant tenderness. She has light-coloured stools and dark urine. Her amylase, bilirubin, uric acid, gamma-glutamyl transferase and liver transaminases are all elevated. Her alkaline phosphatase is 2000 IU/L (30–300 IU/L). The MOST likely diagnosis is

A transplant rejection
B common bile duct stricture
C intrahepatic cholestasis
D primary biliary cirrhosis
E carcinoma of the head of the pancreas

68. A 50-year-old man with insulin dependent diabetes mellitus presents with peripheral oedema and ascites. He has 3+ proteinuria. 24-hour urine collection contains 10 g of protein. His serum albumin is 15 g/L. The MOST likely diagnosis is:

A diabetic nephrosclerosis
B nephrotic syndrome
C uraemia
D interstitial nephritis
E retroperitoneal fibrosis

69. An 80-year-old woman presents with chronic dysphagia and weight loss. She complains of a sensation of a lump in her throat, bad breath, and regurgitation of undigested food. She has a history of recurrent chest infections. She does not smoke or drink alcohol. Physical examination reveals a low BMI and a visible lump on the left side of her neck, which is difficult to define on palpation. The MOST definitive investigation would be

A chest x-ray
B barium meal
C endoscopy and biopsy
D oesophageal motility studies
E indirect laryngoscopy

70. A 19-year-old female presents to Casualty with acute onset of right-sided lower quadrant abdominal pain. She states that the pain is getting worse. She last had unprotected sexual intercourse 2 weeks ago. Her period is due today. Blood pressure is 90/50, pulse 100/min and temperature 37°C. On examination the patient has rebound tenderness in both lower quadrants with guarding. Bowel sounds are absent. On pelvic examination there is tenderness on palpating the cervix and right adnexal discomfort. There are no palpable masses. There is blood in the cervical os. The MOST appropriate management would be

A check urine β-HCG, if positive, resuscitate and crossmatch blood while awaiting urgent gynaecologist referral
B take triple swabs and commence broad-spectrum IV antibiotics
C resuscitate the patient and refer to surgeons for urgent laparotomy
D check urine β-HCG, if positive, send directly to the early pregnancy unit for an urgent transvaginal ultrasound
E check urine β-HCG, if positive, arrange for D & C

71. An 80-year-old man presents with a 2-month history of weakness, dark stools and worsening constipation alternating with episodes of diarrhoea. He has lost a stone in weight. He has a history of diverticular disease and has had 2 myocardial infarctions. Blood tests reveal anaemia, hyponatraemia, hypokalaemia and hypochloraemia. The stool is positive for occult blood. The MOST useful diagnostic investigation is

A chest and abdomen plain x-rays
B mesenteric angiography
C barium enema
D rigid sigmoidoscopy
E barium swallow and meal

72. The following statements regarding cholesterol are correct EXCEPT

A Cholic acid and chenodeoxycholic acid are derived from cholesterol.
B Gallstones are associated with excessive bile salts in relation to the concentrations of cholesterol and phospholipids.
C The rate limiting step in cholesterol synthesis is HMGCoA reductase.
D Plasma cholesterol is raised in thyroid insufficiency.
E Plasma cholesterol is low in cirrhosis.

73. A 40-year-old woman presents with multiple symptoms. She states that for weeks she has felt tired with a loss of appetite. She has intermittent abdominal pain, diarrhoea and has lost half a stone in weight. On examination: temperature 36.5°C, supine BP is 100/60 with a pulse of 90/min; postural hypotension, mild epigastric pain and a pigmented appendicectomy scar. The BEST test to confirm the likely diagnosis is

A serum urea and electrolytes
B short ACTH (synacthen) stimulation test
C random cortisol
D insulin hypoglycaemia test
E adrenal antibodies

74. A 25-year-old woman a month post-partum presents with a painful diffuse thyroid swelling and fever. Her serum thyroxine and ESR are raised. There is no radio-iodine uptake on scanning. The MOST likely diagnosis is

A Hashimoto's disease
B de Quervain's thyroiditis
C Grave's disease
D Reidel's thyroiditis
E multinodular goitre

75. A 30-year-old woman presents with a diffusely enlarged thyroid gland associated with a bruit. Her serum thyroxine is raised and TSH is low. The MOST discriminating investigation to establish the aetiology would be

A ultrasound scan
B fine-needle biopsy
C serum thyroid-stimulating immunoglobulins against TSH receptor
D radio-iodine scan
E thyroid releasing hormone (TRH) test

76. A 50-year-old woman is noted to have a high serum calcium, low-normal phosphate and normal albumin on routine biochemistry test. She is asymptomatic. The MOST useful additional blood test would be

A serum chloride
B serum parathyroid hormone (PTH)
C serum magnesium
D serum urea
E serum alkaline phosphatase

77. A 90-year-old man is noted to have a serum alkaline phosphatase of 1050 IU/L (30–300 IU/L) on routine blood tests. He is asymptomatic. His calcium, phosphate, and PTH levels are normal. The MOST likely diagnosis is

A multiple myeloma
B osteitis deformans
C bone metastases
D hyperparathyroidism
E osteomalacia

78. A 25-year-old obese lady presents with mood swings, acne, secondary amenorrhoea and hirsutism. She has mild lower back pain, which she relates to her weight problem. She smokes 20 cigarettes a day and drinks alcohol at weekends. BP is 125/85 and urine dipstick is negative for glucose. The MOST discriminating blood test is

A serum LH/ FSH ratio and testosterone
B free T4 and TSH
C serum cortisol
D dexamethasone suppression test
E CEA-125

79. The Multiple Endocrine Neoplasia type I syndrome comprises which ONE of the following

A pituitary adenoma, parathyroid hyperplasia and pancreatic islet cell tumour
B phaeochromocytoma, parathyroid hyperplasia and pancreatic islet cell tumour
C medullary carcinoma of the thyroid, phaeochromocytoma, and parathyroid hyperplasia
D phaeochromocytoma, pituitary adenoma, and parathyroid hyperplasia
E pituitary adenoma, phaeochromocytoma, and pancreatic islet cell tumour

80. A 36-year-old woman diagnosed with premature ovarian failure now presents with bone pain. Her serum calcium, phosphate and alkaline phosphatase and urinary calcium are all normal. The MOST likely diagnosis is

A osteomalacia
B osteoporosis
C bone metastasis
D secondary hyperparathyroidism
E multiple myeloma

81. A 50-year-old Middle Eastern woman presents with pain in her thighs. She complains of difficulty in rising from a chair. Her serum calcium is low-normal. Her serum phosphate is reduced and her alkaline phosphatase is raised. X-ray of her pelvis and femurs show translucent 2 mm bands perpendicular to the surface of the bone extending from the cortex inwards in the right femur. The MOST likely diagnosis is

A osteoporosis
B osteomalacia
C Paget's disease
D polymyalgia rheumatica
E multiple myeloma

82. A 45-year-old female underwent mastectomy with axillary clearance 2 years ago. Following this she developed a manic-depressive illness and now presents with excessive thirst and polyuria. Investigations show

Serum sodium	150 mmol/ L
Serum potassium	3.8 mmol/L
Serum calcium	3.1 mmol/L
Random serum glucose	9 mmol/L
Serum urea	6 mmol/L
Serum creatinine	100 μmol/L
Urine osmolality	150 mosm/kg

Following desmopressin, her urine osmolality increases to 250 mosm/kg. The MOST likely cause for her condition is

A metastatic breast carcinoma
B lithium
C pituitary tumour
D diabetes mellitus
E primary polydipsia

83.
Serum sodium	134 mmol/L	pH	7.20
Serum potassium	5.6 mmol/L	pCO_2	3 kPa
Serum chloride	95 mmol/L		
Serum bicarbonate	20 mmol/L		

The above results are ONLY compatible with a diagnosis of

A excessive vomiting
B excessive diarrhoea
C diabetic ketoacidosis
D Addison's disease
E renal tubular disease

84. A 45-year-old woman presents with a 2-month history of fatigue. She smokes 20 cigarettes a day and drinks alcohol at weekends. Her BP is 165/100. Her serum AM cortisol is 800 nmol/L (450-700 nmol/L). Her 24-hour urine collection for urine free cortisol comes back as 1000 nmol/L (<700 nmol/24 hr). Overnight dexamethasone test results in high AM cortisol. However there is some response to high dose dexamethasone. The MOST likely diagnosis is

A ectopic ACTH secretion from small cell carcinoma of the bronchus
B adrenocortical tumour
C Cushing's disease
D alcoholism
E depression

85. A 14-year-old girl with Turner's syndrome presents with short stature. X-rays confirm that the epiphyses have not yet closed. The MOST appropriate management would be

A somatropin
B oestrogen supplementation
C refer for consultation with orthopaedic surgeon for leg-lengthening
D bone scan
E growth hormone levels

86. Causes of transient urinary incontinence include all of the following EXCEPT

A faecal impaction
B atrophic vaginitis
C calcium channel blockers
D tricyclic antidepressant therapy
E delirium

87. Complications of nephrotic syndrome include all of the following EXCEPT

A renal vein thrombosis
B renal artery stenosis
C pneumococcal peritonitis
D hypercholesterolaemia
E hypovolaemia

88. A 30-year-old woman presents with fever, cough and haematuria. She had been in Egypt 2 weeks previously. On examination she has hepatomegaly. Ultrasound shows renal congestion, hydronephrosis and thickened bladder wall but no calcification. The MOST likely diagnosis is

A schistosomiasis haematobium
B schistosomiasis mansoni
C genitourinary tuberculosis
D focal segmental glomerulonephritis
E plasmodium malariae

89. A 30-year-old man presents with acute loin pain and haematuria. He has a history of recurrent urinary tract infections. He states that his father also had kidney problems and had suffered from a bleed in the brain. On examination his BP is 160/100, and he has ballotable large, irregular kidneys and hepatomegaly. The MOST definitive investigation would be:

A kidney-ureter-bladder plain film (KUB)
B excretion urography
C CT scan of the abdomen
D renal ultrasound
E urinalysis and MSU for culture and sensitivities

90. Causes of alopecia include all of the following EXCEPT

A zinc deficiency
B iron deficiency
C nicotinic acid (niacin) deficiency
D polycystic ovaries
E pernicious anaemia

91. A 25-year-old man presents with an intensely pruritic rash over his hands, buttock and penis. The itching is worse at night. He had unprotected sexual intercourse a few days ago. On examination there are delicate scaling areas with threadlike linear tracks on the sides of his hands, palms and buttocks. His penis is covered with large, pruritic, crusted papules and nodules. The BEST way to make a diagnosis is

A microscopic examination for mite and eggs on a potassium hydroxide preparation of scraping from tracks
B clear tape removal and microscopic examination for adherent eggs
C VDRL
D skin biopsy with immunofluorescent staining
E direct inspection for multiple eggs and lice

92. Lichen planus lesions are associated with all of the following EXCEPT

    A pre-malignancy
    B myasthenia gravis
    C thiazides
    D graft-vs-host disease
    E Koebner phenomenon

93. A 20-year-old woman complains of fever, arthralgia and a rash. On examination she is found to have oral aphthous ulcers and pleomorphic erythematous bullous eruptions with concentric rings on her forearms and legs. She is not taking any medication. The MOST likely diagnosis

    A erythema multiforme
    B erythema nodosum
    C erythema marginatum
    D pemphigus vulgaris
    E Behçet's disease

94. A 30-year-old female presents with a 2-week history of a non-pruritic rash on her trunk, back and upper arms. It started with a single patch on her left scapula. She denies fever or taking medication. On examination she has ovoid erythematous macules with delicate while scaling collars arranged according to the lines of cleavage of the skin. The patch on her left scapula is the largest. Her face, lower arms and lower extremities are spared. The MOST likely cause is

    A secondary syphilis
    B guttate psoriasis
    C nummular eczematous dermatitis
    D pityriasis rosea
    E erythema chronicum migrans

95. A 30-year-old HIV-positive man on anti-tuberculosis chemotherapy presents with gradual loss of vision in his right eye. On examination he has a relative afferent pupillary defect and loss of red colour vision. The optic disc is slightly swollen. The MOST likely diagnosis is

    A TB meningitis
    B macular degeneration
    C optic neuritis
    D CMV retinitis
    E optic atrophy

96. A 25-year-old HIV positive man presents with two weeks of worsening drowsiness. On examination he has cervical lymphadenopathy and has bilateral upgoing plantar reflexes. CT scan of the head shows cerebral calcifications and ring lesions. The MOST likely diagnosis is

A cerebral toxoplasmosis
B cerebral abscess
C lymphoma
D cryptococcus meningitis
E tuberculosis

97. A 20-year-old woman presents with copious foul-smelling green vaginal discharge and sore throat. She last had unprotected oral and vaginal sexual intercourse 2 days ago. She is 3 months pregnant. The MOST appropriate treatment is

A oral ciprofloxacin 500 mg stat
B oral amoxycillin 3 g stat
C doxycycline 100 mg bd for 5 days
D metronidazole 400 mg tds for 5 days
E cefoxitin 2 g IM + probenecid 1 g by mouth

98. A 22-year-old female presents with frothy gray vaginal discharge. She states that she last had unprotected sexual intercourse 2 weeks ago. The vaginal discharge is noted to have a pH of 5 and emits a fishy odour on alkalinisation with potassium hydroxide. The MOST appropriate treatment is

A oral ciprofloxacin 500 mg stat
B doxycycline 100 mg o bd for 5 days
C metronidazole 400 mg o tds for 5 days
D none as it is not a sexually-transmitted disease
E clotrimazole pessaries

99. A 30-year-old man presents with right ocular pain and blurring of vision and purulent green urethral discharge. He had unprotected sex a week ago. The MOST likely diagnosis is

A chlamydia trachomatis
B Reiter's syndrome
C gonococcal urethritis
D syphilis
E trichomonas

100. A 25-year-old homosexual man presents with swinging fever and rigors. He denies intravenous drug abuse and is not on any medication. On examination he has a pansystolic murmur at the lower sternal border. He is also noted to have pharyngitis and mild proctitis. The MOST likely organism responsible for his presumed infective endocarditis is

A Streptococcus faecalis
B Candida albicans
C Neisseria gonorrhoea
D Streptococcus viridans
E Streptococcus pneumoniae

Answers to Paper Five BOFs

Criterion Referencing Marks

* – 25–50% of candidates expected to get correct
** – 50–75% of candidates expected to get correct
*** – 75–100% of candidates expected to get correct

The notional PASS MARK is 76%

1. E ***

2. E **

3. D **

4. D ***

5. E **

6. B ** The patient has blackwater fever, a complication of infection with P. falciparum.

7. B ** A patient with jaundice and acute renal failure should raise suspicion of leptospirosis (Weil's disease).

8. B ***

9. C *** Cryoprecipitate does not contain Factor IX.

10. A ***

11. C *** Blood replacement contains excess citrate associated with hypocalcaemia.

12. E ***

13. A ** C3a and C5a are chemical mediators of increased vascular permeability.

14. E *** Post-splenectomy may be associated with early thombocytosis.

15. D ***

16. B ***

17. B ***

18. E ***

19. B ** TCA overdose is associated with fits, arrhythmias, urinary retention and pupillary dilation. Barbiturate poisoning is also associated with pupillary dilation but not with arrhythmias.

20. D ***

21. A **

22. E **

23. C **

24. E * Sodium valproate is associated with inhibition of platelet aggregation and thrombocytopaenia.

25. B ***

26. D ***

27. C **

28. D ** The boy's antinuclear antibodies are positive which is associated with the development of iritis and may lead ultimately to blindness.

29. B ***

30. E ***

31. E ***

32. A ***

33. A ***

34. C *** Pulseless ventricular tachycardia is a shockable rhythm.

35. C ***

36. E ***

37. B *** Cystic fibrosis is associated with absent vas deferens and epididymis.

38. A ** PEEP is associated with decreased cardiac output.

39. D ***

40. A ***

41. A ***

42. B ***

43. C ***

44. D *

45. B *

46. B ** The area of cellulitis in this patient also coincides with the drainage area of the midbrain. Consequently, the patient is at risk of cavernous sinus thrombosis.

47. B ***

48. C *** Devic syndrome is a form of multiple sclerosis.

49. A ***

50. B **

51. D ** This patient has bilateral acoustic neuromas.

52. E *** Eaton–Lambert syndrome is associated with small-cell carcinoma of the bronchus.

53. B **

54. D **

55. C ***

56. A ** The cornea stains like a dendritic tree with sharp-borders around the ulcer.

57. B ** Topical application of LA is contraindicated as the patient will be tempted to rub her eye and extend the corneal abrasion. Double padding is advised to prevent any interference with corneal healing.

58. D ** Caffeine intoxication and not withdrawal may mimic panic disorder.

59. E **

60. D *** Bulimics have irregular periods. Anorexics have no periods.

61. A ***

62. D ***

63. D ***

64. A ***

65. D **

66. A *** This patient has irritable bowel syndrome which may be treated with an antispasmodic prn.

67. B **

68. B ***

69. B ***

70. A *** The initial management should be to resuscitate the patient and determine whether she is pregnant. Sending a patient in her condition straight up to the early pregnancy unit without IV access and a drip is ill-advised. She will of course require an urgent transvaginal ultrasound to exclude ectopic pregnancy.

71. C ** Colonoscopy, if patient is fit enough, would be the best choice but has not been offered as an option!

72. B ***

73. B ***

74. B ***

75. C ***

76. B ***

77. B ***

78. A ***

79. A ***

80. B ***

81. B ***

82. A **

83. C ** The results indicate a metabolic acidosis with an increased anion gap.

84. C ***

85. A * Somatropin is a synthetic human growth hormone produced by recombinant DNA technique and has now replaced somatotrophin (HGH).

86. D ** TCA's have been used to treat urinary incontinence.

87. B ** The patient is at risk of renal vein thrombosis.

88. A **

89. D ***

90. C **

91. A **

92. A **

93. A ** Herpes simplex virus is a common cause of erythema multiforme.

94. D **

95. C * This patient is taking ethambutol as part of his anti-tuberculosis therapy. Ethambutol is associated with optic neuritis.

96. A ***

97. B ***

98. C * Gardnerella is not a STD and usually results from excessive douching and bubble baths but nonetheless is treated with metronidazole for overgrowth of anaerobic bacteria.

99. C *** This patient has iritis and purulent urethritis suggestive of GC.

100. C ***

MRCP Paper Six MCQs

Questions

1. The following statements are correct

   A A lesion of the oculomotor nerve would result in ptosis.
   B A lesion of the facial nerve would result in diminished corneal reflex.
   C A lesion of the trigeminal nerve would result in enhanced jaw jerk reflex.
   D An UMN lesion of the hypoglossal nerve would result in deviation of the tongue towards the side of the lesion.
   E A lesion of the spinal accessory nerve would result in a winged scapula.

2. The uptake of oxygen by haemoglobin

   A is increased by a rise in temperature
   B is decreased by a fall in pH
   C is increased by a rise in 2,3-DPG
   D is increased by the presence of carbon monoxide
   E is increased by the presence of fetal haemoglobin

3. Berry aneurysm

   A is a rare cause of subarachnoid haemorrhage
   B may result in a communicating hydrocephalus
   C is associated with polycystic kidney disease
   D is associated with coarctation of the aorta
   E is associated with Type III collagen deficiency

4. Causes of hypokalaemia include

   A intestinal fistula
   B metabolic acidosis
   C pyloric stenosis
   D amiloride-frusemide combination therapy
   E massive blood transfusion

5. Iron

   A in the ferric state is reduced before it can be absorbed
   B absorption is hindered by ascorbic acid
   C absorption is hindered by alcohol
   D poisoning is treated with desferrioxamine
   E deficiency is associated with decreased total iron binding capacity

6. In iron metabolism

   A 70% of dietary iron is absorbed
   B Iron absorption occurs mainly in the ileum
   C Excess iron in the intestinal cell is converted to ferritin
   D Iron is transported in the plasma bound to apoferritin
   E Iron is stored in the tissues as ferritin

7. The following statements regarding carbon dioxide are true

   A Arterial CO_2 pressure falls during sleep.
   B It is 30 times more soluble than oxygen.
   C It may frequently be affected by diffusion disorders.
   D A decrease in carbon dioxide pressure stimulates the carotid bodies.
   E Central chemoreceptors are not sensitive to carbon dioxide.

8. Commensal bacteria are found in the

   A urethra
   B vagina
   C external auditory meatus
   D nasal vestibule
   E bronchus

9. Lymphokines

   A are proteins produced by B-lymphocytes
   B are important in eosinophil activation
   C are important in immune complex disease
   D aid in elimination of toxoplasma gondii
   E stimulate the proliferation of B and T cells

10. IgG antibodies

   A are the first antibody to appear in the immune response
   B form the highest proportion of the serum immunoglobulins
   C can fix complement via the alternative pathway
   D can cross placenta
   E have the longest half-life of all the immunoglobulins

11. The following statements regarding plasma autoantibodies are correct

    A Antinuclear antibody is found in the majority of patients with juvenile rheumatoid arthritis.
    B Rheumatoid factor is positive in Still's disease.
    C ANCA is positive in 95% of cases of Wegener's granulomatosis.
    D Sjogren's syndrome is characterised by the presence of anti-rho antibodies.
    E Antibody to mitochondria is found in most cases of primary biliary cirrhosis.

12. Cell-mediated immunity

    A is usually short-lasting
    B can be detected by skin test
    C is mediated by B-lymphocytes
    D is based on delayed hypersensitivity
    E is associated with decreased macrophage activity

13. Lymphocytosis is seen in infection of

    A toxoplasmosis
    B Legionnaire's disease
    C infectious mononucleosis
    D cytomegalovirus
    E rubella

14. The following pairs are correctly matched

    A chronic otitis externa – moraxella catarrhalis
    B Lyme disease – Borrelia burgdorferi
    C gas gangrene – Clostridium perfringens
    D abattoir worker – Bacillus anthracis
    E traveller's diarrhoea – Vibrio cholerae

15. Infection with the following organisms typically manifest with offensive vaginal discharge

    A chlamydia trachomatis
    B neisseria gonorrhoea
    C trichomonas vaginalis
    D gardnerella vaginalis
    E treponema pallidum

16. A 40-year-old man presents with fever, headache, and vomiting. His lumbar puncture reveals $20/mm^3$ mononuclear cells, 2 g/l of protein and glucose of half the plasma level. There are no organisms in the smear. Appropriate treatment options include

   A amphotericin B and flucytosine
   B cefotaxime
   C rifampicin, ethambutol, izoniazid and pyrazinamide
   D withhold treatment till culture results are back
   E benzylpenicillin

17. Recognised manifestastions of chlamydia trachomatis infection include

   A inclusion conjunctivitis
   B ophthalmia neonatorum
   C lymphogranuloma venereum
   D subacute bacterial endocarditis
   E vulval elephantiasis

18. Features of Lyme disease include

   A erythema chronicum migrans
   B lymphocytic meningoradiculitis (Bannwarth's syndrome)
   C facial nerve palsy
   D myositis
   E renal failure

19. Prolonged bleeding time is seen in

   A severe aplastic anaemia
   B haemophilia A
   C Von Willebrand's disease
   D immune thrombocytopaenic purpura
   E Henoch–Schönlein purpura

20. Primary (autoimmune) thrombocytopaenic purpura is associated with

   A splenomegaly
   B decreased number of megakaryocytes in the bone marrow
   C menorrhagia
   D shortened platelet survival time
   E transfused platelets surviving longer than the patient's own

21. Aciclovir

    A is an ester of valaciclovir
    B eradicates the herpes virus
    C is recommended for treatment of condylomata accuminatum
    D is effective only if commenced at the onset of the infection
    E may be used topically to treat dendritic corneal ulcers

22. A less than 50% five-year survival is expected despite management and treatment of the following conditions

    A acute lymphoblastic leukaemia L3 subtype presenting in an 8-year-old boy
    B chronic lymphocytic leukaemia presenting in a 60-year-old man with a Hb of 11g/dL and a white cell count of 16×10^9/L and no enlarged lymph nodes or organs
    C mixed cellularity Hodgkin's lymphoma presenting in a 25-year-old woman with an enlarged painless cervical lymph node
    D multiple myeloma presenting in a 70-year-old with a urea of 11 mmol/L and a Hb of 7 g/dL.
    E diffuse large-cleaved grade Non-Hodgkin's lymphoma presenting in a 60-year-old man with constitutional symptoms

23. Basal cell carcinoma

    A often metastasizes
    B is associated with Bowen's disease
    C is commoner in white than black skins
    D is commonly sited on the upper lip
    E is the commonest skin cancer

24. Causes of secondary polycythaemia include

    A renal cell carcinoma
    B high altitudes
    C hydronephrosis
    D cerebellar haemangioblastoma
    E cor pulmonale

25. In hereditary spherocytosis

    A inheritance is autosomal recessive
    B there is an intrinsic defect in the erythrocyte membrane spectrin
    C presentation may be with jaundice
    D there is increased osmotic fragility
    E there is a positive Coombs' test

26. The following statements are correct

   A Beta-thalassaemia is characterised by suppression of the beta chain synthesis.
   B Sickle cell anaemia is caused by the substitution of glutamine for valine at position 6 of the beta chain of haemoglobin.
   C Heinz bodies may be seen in alpha-thalassaemia.
   D Most patients with beta-thalassaemia minor die by the third decade.
   E Target cells are not seen in thalassaemia minor.

27. Prothrombin time is increased in

   A obstructive jaundice
   B heparin therapy
   C von Willebrand's disease
   D hepatocellular disease
   E disseminated intravascular coagulation

28. The following are absolute contraindications to the combined oral contraceptive pill in a 30-year-old

   A ergotamine
   B smoking 30 cigarettes per day
   C migraine without focal aura
   D systemic lupus erythematosus
   E blood pressure of 140/90

29. Features of pulmonary stenosis include

   A widely split S1
   B prominent a waves in JVP
   C RV heave
   D systolic ejection murmur loudest to the left of the upper sternum border
   E early diastolic (Graham Steel) murmur

30. Systemic hypertension is seen in

   A diabetes mellitus
   B Conn's syndrome
   C phaeochromocytoma
   D hyperparathyroidism
   E acromegaly

31. Myocardial infarction is a recognised complication of

    A polyarteritis nodosa
    B Wegener's granulomatosis
    C Takayasu's arteritis
    D rheumatic fever
    E subacute bacterial endocarditis

32. Clinical features associated with acute infective endocarditis include

    A Heberden's nodes
    B palmar macules (Janeway lesions)
    C nail pitting
    D small grey plaques raised from the interpalpebral conjunctiva (Bitot's spots)
    E splenomegaly

33. The following statements regarding findings in mitral stenosis are correct:

    A There is increased pulmonary capillary wedge pressure.
    B There is an early diastolic murmur.
    C Opening snap occurs in early diastole.
    D Echocardiogram is sufficiently accurate to allow surgical management to be considered.
    E Atrial fibrillation is rarely present.

34. In paroxysmal supra-ventricular tachycardia

    A the heart rate is between 150 and 250 beats per minute
    B the P to QRS ratio is not 1:1
    C IV adenosine is contraindicated in patients with asthma
    D IV verapamil should be given if there is a recent history of use of β-blockers
    E DC cardioversion is ineffective

35. Excess digitalis is associated with the following ECG changes

    A paroxysmal atrial tachycardia with block
    B nodal tachycardia with AV dissociation
    C short QT interval
    D wide notched P
    E ST elevation in all leads

36. The following cutaneous markers of malignancy are correctly paired

   A erythema gyuratum repens – carcinoma of the bronchus
   B necrolytic migratory erythema – glucagonoma
   C acquired icthyosis – lymphoma
   D thrombophlebitis migrans – carcinoma of the pancreas
   E circumoral pigmentation – Peutz–Jegher syndrome

37. Causes of low-output heart failure include

   A Trypanosoma Cruzii infection (Chagas' disease)
   B Paget's disease
   C arteriovenous malformation
   D pregnancy
   E aortic stenosis

38. Asbestosis is associated with

   A mesothelioma
   B pleural plaques
   C pulmonary eosinophilia
   D interstitial fibrosis
   E increased risk of developing tuberculosis

39. The following statements regarding bronchogenic carcinoma are correct

   A Uranium exposure is a recognised risk factor.
   B Large cell carcinoma is associated with paraneoplastic syndromes.
   C Adenocarcinoma is the most common type of bronchogenic carcinoma.
   D Small (oat) cell carcinoma occurs in the peripheral lung fields.
   E Hypercalcaemia is associated with squamous cell carcinoma.

40. The following statements are correct

   A The response to high ventilation/perfusion (V/Q) ratio is vasoconstriction.
   B In normal lungs in the upright position, V/Q ratio is lower in the lower lobes.
   C In pulmonary embolism without infarction V/Q ratio is high.
   D V/Q ratio is zero if the bronchus is occluded.
   E An increased V/Q ratio represents increased physiological dead space.

41. The following statements regarding asthma are correct

    A It may present with nocturnal coughing.
    B It may be associated with pulsus paradoxus.
    C Patients who are symptomatic in spite of treatment with β-2 agonists should be commenced on oral corticosteroids.
    D If the PEFR is <150 L/min, the patient should be admitted to hospital.
    E Ketotifen is an anti-cholinergic bronchodilator.

42. Pulmonary oedema is a complication of

    A blood transfusion
    B chronic bronchitis
    C mitral stenosis
    D nephrotic syndrome
    E aspiration of pleural effusion

43. Characteristic findings in subacute combined degeneration of the cord are

    A dementia
    B positive Babinski sign
    C absent knee jerk reflex
    D intact vibration sense
    E optic atrophy

44. Raised protein and IgG in the CSF at lumbar puncture is associated with

    A meningococcal meningitis
    B tuberculous meningitis
    C pneumococcal meningitis
    D multiple sclerosis
    E viral meningitis

45. Depression is commonly associated with

    A anhedonia
    B dysphoria
    C depersonalisation
    D early morning awakening
    E flat affect

46. Organic causes of dementia include

A pernicious anaemia
B extradural haematoma
C primary syphilis
D phaeochromocytoma
E Addison's disease

47. Causes of portal vein thrombosis include

A pyelophlebitis after acute appendicitis
B schistosomiasis
C neonatal exchange transfusion
D Budd–Chiari syndrome
E tricuspid valve incompetence

48. Oesophageal cancer is associated with

A Barrett's oesophagus
B achalasia
C Crohn's disease
D pernicious anaemia
E coeliac disease

49. The following statements regarding oral hypoglycaemics are correct

A Metformin is a biguanide that may cause metabolic alkalosis.
B Chlorpropramide has the least number of side-effects of the sulfonylureas.
C Sulphonylureas act by increasing insulin secretion.
D Gliblenclamide is associated with facial flushing after drinking alcohol.
E Repaglinide may be used in conjunction with metformin.

50. Severe diabetic ketoacidosis may present with

A hypoventilation
B hyperkalaemia
C an elevated white cell count in the absence of infection
D ketonuria
E abdominal pain

51. Accidental hypothermia is associated with

A a core (rectal) temperature of <36 degrees celsius
B pancreatitis
C pneumonia
D intra-vascular haemolysis
E atrial fibrillation

52. The following statements regarding diabetes insipidus (DI) are correct

   A It is excluded if the water deprivation test reveals a first morning urine osmolality <600 mosm/kg.
   B In nephrogenic DI, the urine osmolality increases by >60% following desmopressin.
   C In cranial DI, there is diminished synthesis of ADH in the posterior pituitary.
   D Sarcoidosis may cause nephrogenic DI.
   E Pregnancy aggravates untreated DI.

53. The following statements regarding primary hyperparathyroidism are correct

   A It may present with peptic ulcer.
   B Hyperphosphataemia is common.
   C Hypercalcaemia is resistant to suppression by steroids.
   D Plasma chloride is decreased.
   E Parathyroid adenomata may be present in the upper mediastinum.

54. The following statements regarding vitamin D are correct

   A Deficiency is associated with osteoporosis.
   B Deficiency is associated with delayed bone fracture healing.
   C Deficiency is associated with secondary hyperparathyroidism.
   D It is produced in the skin as cholecalciferol.
   E Hypocalcaemia stimulates $1,25 (OH)_2 D3$ (calcitriol) production.

55. Renal papillary necrosis is a recognised complication of

   A diabetes mellitus
   B sickle cell trait
   C phenacetin
   D dihydrocodeine
   E Sjogren's syndrome

56. The following statements regarding renal calculi are correct

   A Calcium phosphate stones are the most common type.
   B Sarcoidosis is associated with renal calculi.
   C Crohn's disease is associated with hyperoxaluria.
   D Proteus mirabilis infection gives rise to staghorn calculi.
   E Uric acid stones imply hyperuricaemia.

57. Bladder tumours

   A present with painful haematuria
   B when associated with schistosomiasis are transitional cell carcinomas
   C are 50 times as common as those of the renal pelvis or ureter
   D are associated with alcohol abuse
   E are treated with cyclophosphamide

58. In polymyalgia rheumatica

   A the dramatic response to prednisolone is a diagnostic feature
   B serum creatinine kinase is normal
   C serum ESR is elevated
   D rheumatoid factor is positive
   E serum alkaline phosphatase may be raised

59. Chondrocalcinosis (calcification of the joint cartilage) is seen in

   A pyrophosphate arthropathy
   B haemophilia
   C primary hyperparathyroidism
   D ankylosing spondylitis
   E haemochromatosis

60. Non-gonococcal urethritis

   A is less common than gonococcal urethritis
   B in women is typically asymptomatic
   C is treated with doxycycline
   D may be associated with Reiter's syndrome
   E may infect the pharynx and rectum

Answers to Paper Six MCQs

Criterion Referencing Marks

*   – 25–50% of candidates expected to get correct
**   – 50–75% of candidates expected to get correct
***   – 75–100% of candidates expected to get correct

The notional PASS MARK is 228/300 or 76%

---

1. TFFFF *** A lesion of the trigeminal nerve would result in diminished corneal and jaw jerk reflexes. A lesion of the long thoracic nerve results in a winged scapula. A LMN lesion of the hypoglossal nerve would result in deviation of the tongue towards the side of the lesion. An UMN lesion would have the opposite effect.

2. FTFFT ** The uptake of oxygen by haemoglobin is decreased by a rise in temperature, a fall in pH, a rise in 2,3-DPG, and by the presence of CO.

3. FTTTF ** Berry aneuryms are the most common cause of nontraumatic subarachnoid haemorrhage.

4. TFTFF *** Metabolic acidosis, amiloride (K-sparing) diuretic and massive blood transfusion are associated with hyperkalaemia.

5. TFFTF ** Ascorbic acid, alcohol and gastric acid all facilitate iron absorption. TIBC increase in iron deficiency anaemia.

6. FFTFT ** Only 10% of iron in one's daily diet is absorbed. Absorption takes place in the duodenum and jejunum. Iron is transported in plasma bound to transferrin.

7. FTFFF ** Carbon dioxide is extremely soluble and is rarely affected by diffusion difficulties. An increase in carbon dioxide pressures triggers both carotid bodies (peripheral chemoreceptors) and central chemoreceptors.

8. FTTTF *** Commensals are normal bacterial flora.

9. TTFTF ** Lymphokines are produced by both activated T and B-lymphocytes. Interleukin 1 and 2 stimulate the proliferation of B and T cells.

10. FTFTF ** IgM is the first antibody in the immune response. IgE has the longest half-life.

11. TFTTT ** Rheumatoid factor is rarely positive in Still's disease.

12. FTFTF *** Cell-mediated immunity is long-lasting and is mediated by T-lymphocytes. There is an increase in macrophage activity.

13. TFTTT **

14. FTTTF ** Chronic otitis externa is associated with infection with pseudomonas pyocaneus. E. coli is associated with traveller's diarrhoea.

15. FTTTF **

16. FFTFF ***

17. TFTFT * Ophthalmia neonatorum is associated with N. gonorrhoea infection. Chlamydia psittacosis may give rise to SBE.

18. TTTFF ** Lyme disease is a tick-borne disease caused by Borrelia burgdorferi. It is also associated with cardiac conduction abnormalities in 10% of cases.

19. TFTTF *** Bleeding time is prolonged with platelet disorders.

20. FFTTF ** Splenomegaly is rarely seen in ITP, though splenectomy may be curative. There is an increased number of megakaryocytes. Menorrhagia, epistaxis, and easy bruising are all common presentations. Transfused platelets survive no longer than the patient's own. ITP is associated with a prolonged bleeding time secondary to excess destruction of platelets.

21. FFFTT ** Valaciclovir is an ester and prodrug of aciclovir. Aciclovir is active against the herpes virus but does not eradicate the virus. It is recommended for treatment of herpes simplex and varicella-zoster infections.

22. TFFTT * Poor prognosis in ALL is associated with subtype L3, male sex and age >10 years. The example of CLL is classified as Stage 0 and has a good prognosis. Mixed cellularity grade Hodgkin's lymphoma has a good prognosis. She also has stage 0 disease. Lymphocyte depleted grade has the worst prognosis. Multiple myeloma has a 50% 2-year survival made worse if the urea is >10 mmol/L and the Hb is <7.5g/dL. Diffuse large-cleaved grade NHL is an intermediate grade with a 35% 5-year survival. Associated constitutional symptoms offer a worse prognosis.

23. FFFFT *** Basal cell carcinoma rarely metastasises. Squamous cell carcinoma is associated with Bowen's disease, Marjolin ulcers, actinic keratoses and occur on the upper lip.

24. TTTTT ** Other causes include chronic lung disease and cyanotic congenital heart disease.

25. FTTTF *** Hereditary spherocytosis is an autosomal dominant inherited condition. It may present with jaundice (cholelithiasis) or haemolytic crisis (i.e. parvovirus infection) with raised serum bilirubin and urinary urobilinogen. Following splenectomy, the spherocytosis is reduced. The Coombs' test is negative.

26. TFTFF *** Sickle cell disease is caused by the vice versa substitution, i.e. valine for glutamine at position 6. Heinz bodies are seen in splenectomised patients with alpha-thalassaemia. Target cells are seen in both forms of thalassaemia. Beta-thalassaemia major is associated with a poor prognosis not thalassaemia minor.

27. TFFTT *** PT is increased in warfarin therapy.

28. TFFTF ** Absolute contraindications also include smoking >40 cigs/day, age >50, blood pressure >160/100, weight >39 kg/m^2, migraine attacks with focal aura, attacks requiring ergotamine treatment.

29. FTTTF *** Pulmonary stenosis is associated with a widely-split S2. The Graham Steel murmur is a decrescendo murmur at early diastole heard best at the left sternal edge and is associated with pulmonary regurgitation.

30. FTTTT ***

31. TFFFF *** Kawasaki's disease is the childhood variant of polyarteritis nodosa.

32. FTFFT *** Infective endocarditis is associated with Osler's nodes, Roth spots, finger clubbing, splinter haemorrhages and petechial haemorrhages.

33. TFTTF *** Mitral stenosis is associated with a mid-diastolic murmur. It is frequently complicated by atrial fibrillation.

34. TFTFF *** PSVT has a P to QRS ratio of 1:1. Adenosine may precipitate bronchospasm in asthmatics. Verapamil is contraindicated in the presence of β-blockers.

35. TTFFF ** Excess digitalis is associated with ST depression and scooping diffusely in all leads.

36. TTTTT ***

37. TFFFT *** Paget's disease, AV malformation, pregnancy and hyperthyroidism are examples of causes of high-output cardiac failure.

38. TTFTF *** Asbestosis is associated with increased lung carcinoma and mesothelioma 20 years after exposure. Silicosis is associated with increased risk of tuberculosis.

39. TFFFT *** Small (oat) cell carcinoma is associated with paraneoplastic syndromes and occurs centrally. Squamous cell carcinoma is the most common type of bronchogenic carcinoma and is frequently associated with hypercalcaemia.

40. FTFTT * The response to a high V/Q ratio is bronchoconstriction. Septal defects result in abnormal left to right shunts.

41. TTFTF *** Inhaled corticosteroids are the next line of therapy after β-2 adrenergic agonists. Ipratropium bromide is an effective anti-cholinergic bronchodilator. Ketotifen is an anti-histamine.

42. TFTTT ***

43. FTTFF ** Subacute combined degeneration of the cord is also associated with pernicious anaemia, vitiligo, Addison's disease, and thyroid disease. Vibration sense is absent, with both knee and ankle jerk reflexes.

44. FFFTF ** IgG is present in the CSF of 70% of patients with MS.

45. TTFTF ***

46. TFFFF *** Dementia may be associated with chronic subdural haematoma and tertiary syphilis. Addison's disease may be associated with depression.

47. TFTFF *** Portal vein thrombosis is a cause of prehepatic portal hypertension. Schistosomiasis is a hepatic cause of portal hypertension. Budd–Chiari syndrome and tricuspid valve incompetence are post-hepatic causes of portal hypertension.

48. TTFFT ***

49. FFTFT *** Metformin may cause lactic acidosis. Chlorpropamide has the most number of side-effects of the sulfonylureas and therefore is no longer recommended by the BNF. Chlorpropamide and not gliblenclamide is associated with facial flushing. Repaglinide may be used solo or in conjunction with metformin in NIDDM that is not responding to diet and exercise.

50. FFTTT *** Severe ketoacidosis is associated with potassium depletion, though blood levels may be raised initially and a plasma glucose of >14 mmol/L. Beware as ketonuria may occur in the presence of a normal glucose.

51. FTTFT ** Hypothermia is defined as a core temperature of <35 degrees celsius. It may be associated with hypothyroidism, alcoholism, Parkinson's disease, and may be complicated by acute renal failure, cardiac arrhythmias, pneumonia and pancreatitis.

52. FFFFT ** DI is excluded if the first morning urine osmolality >800 mosm/kg. In nephrogenic DI, the urine osmolality increases by <45% following desmopressin. ADH is secreted from the posterior pituitary gland and not the anterior gland. Sarcoidosis is a cause of cranial DI. Pregnancy aggravates untreated DI.

53. TFTFT *** Hypophosphataemia is common in hyperparathyroidism. Plasma chloride is increased. Ectopic parathyroids may occur in the neck or upper mediastinum.

54. FTTTT *** Vitamin D deficiency is associated with osteomalacia. It is produced in the skin as cholecalciferol and converted to 25 (OH$_2$) D3 in the liver and then to 1,25 (OH$_2$) D3 in the kidney. Calcitriol stimulates calcium and phosphate absorption from the gut in response to hypocalcaemia or hypophosphataemia.

55. TTTFT ***

56. FTTTF *** Calcium oxalate stones are the most common type of renal calculi. Uric acid stones present in acidic urine and are not always associated with hyperuricaemia (gout).

57. FFTFF *** Bladder carcinoma usually presents with painless haematuria. Schistosomiasis is associated with squamous cell carcinoma of the bladder. Bladder carcinoma is linked to smoking and not alcohol. Cyclophosphamide and phenacetin have been linked to bladder cancer.

58. TTTFT *** In PMR, the rheumatoid factor is negative. False positives may occur in elderly women.

59. TTTFT **

60. FTTTF *** NGU is more common than GC. It may be associated with Reiter's syndrome (keratoderma blenorrhagica, urethritis, conjunctivitis and seronegative arthritis).

In these questions candidates must select one answer only

Questions

1. A 20-year-old woman presents with a temperature of 40°C and a week of bloody diarrhoea. She looks unwell and dehydrated. She has been taking erythromycin for 3 months for acne. She has not travelled abroad, and no one else in the family is unwell. Gram-stain of stool show Gram-positive bacilli. The MOST appropriate treatment for her would be

   A IV vancomycin
   B oral metronidazole
   C oral ciprofloxacin
   D oral co-trimoxazole
   E oral chloramphenicol

2. A 20-year-old man back from hitchhiking through South America a fortnight ago now presents with explosive watery foul-smelling diarrhoea and weight loss. On examination he has abdominal distension. His stools are greasy and contain mucos. The MOST likely diagnosis is

   A shigella dysentery
   B giardiasis
   C amoebic dysentery
   D Crohn's disease
   E cystic fibrosis

3. A 24-year-old male living in New England (North-East USA) presents with unilateral facial nerve palsy. He also complains of malaise, neck stiffness, joint pain and a distinctive rash on his leg. The rash started out as a small papule and is now a red ring, 5 cm across with a faded centre. On examination he is also noted to have a pericardial friction rub. The MOST likely diagnosis is

   A Guillain–Barré syndrome
   B sarcoidosis
   C Rocky Mountain spotted fever
   D Lyme disease
   E leprosy

4. The rash is MOST likely

   A erythema marginatum
   B erythema chronicum migrans
   C erythema multiforme
   D erythema nodosum
   E granuloma annulare

5. A 30-year-old eight week pregnant woman is found to be HIV positive with a viral load of 20,000 and a CD4 count of 300. The MOST appropriate management would be

   A arrange for therapeutic abortion
   B commence therapy with two reverse transcriptase inhibitors (RTI) and one protease inhibitor
   C repeat tests in 3 months
   D commence therapy with two non-nucleoside reverse transcriptase inhibitors (NNRTI) and one protease inhibitor
   E commence therapy with one RTI, one NNRTI and one protease inhibitor

6. A 24-year-old African man presents to Casualty with acute onset of fever, vomiting, jaundice and dark brown-black urine. He had been travelling through Africa 6 weeks ago and had taken chloroquine prophylaxis. He is not taking any medication now. On examination he has irregular fever patterns and BP 100/60. There is hepatosplenomegaly, hypertonia and hyper-reflexia. Serum urea and creatinine are markedly elevated and haemoglobinuria is present. The MOST useful investigation is

   A thin and thick Giemsa-stained blood smears
   B enzyme assay for glucose-6-phosphate dehydrogenase deficiency
   C acid-fast staining of stool
   D hepatitis A, B and C virology
   E Yellow Fever serology

7. A 30-year-old man presents with cerebellar ataxia a week after eruption of a generalised rash with vesicles. Smear demonstrates multi-nucleated giant cells. The MOST likely diagnosis is

   A Herpes zoster oticus (Ramsay Hunt syndrome)
   B Herpes simplex encephalitis
   C varicella zoster
   D tuberculosis
   E neurosyphilis

8. A 30-year-old HIV-positive male presents with seizures. The MOST likely infective cause is

   A toxoplasmosis
   B cytomegalovirus
   C cryptosporidium
   D tuberculosis
   E pneumocystis

9. A 50-year-old female complains of fever, vomiting, abdominal pain and diarrhoea. She dined alone at a restaurant 12 hours ago and had eaten chicken curry and drunk lager and water. Blood tests show

Serum sodium	134 mmol/L
Serum potassium	2.0 mmol/L
Serum chloride	105 mmol/L
Serum bicarbonate	30 mmol/L

   The BEST immediate management would be

   A admit for IV hydration and IV potassium replacement at 20 mmol/h
   B treat as outpatient with oral fluids, send stool for culture and sensitivities and notify local Public Health Doctor
   C send stool for culture and sensitivities and encourage fluid intake as an outpatient until sensitivities return
   D encourage oral fluid intake and prescribe erythromycin for presumed campylobacter gastroenteritis
   E encourage oral fluid intake and prescribe ciprofloxacin for presumed salmonella gastroenteritis

10. A 50-year-old man with known liver disease presents with fever, abdominal pain and distension. On examination he has a tender abdomen with shifting dullness. Diagnostic aspirations show elevated neutrophils and Gram-negative rods. The MOST likely organism is

    A Klebiella sp.
    B Escherischia coli
    C Pesudomonas aeruginosa
    D Bacteriodes fragilis
    E Streptococcus pneumonia

11. A 20-year-old African male presents with jaundice and acute short-ness of breath. He had been taking primaquine. His blood tests show raised serum bilirubin, reduced serum haptoglobin and anaemia. The blood film shows Heinz bodies and reticulocytosis. He also has haemoglobinuria and increased urinary urobilinogen. The MOST likely diagnosis is

A glucose-6-phosphate dehydrogenase deficiency
B sickle cell anaemia
C paroxysmal nocturnal haemoglobinuria
D pyruvate kinase deficiency
E autoimmune haemolytic anaemia

12. A 35-year-old female presents with a 1-month history of a painless firm but mobile 2-cm lump in the upper outer quadrant of her breast. No other abnormalities detected. The initial investigation should be

A mammogram
B ultrasound
C fine-needle aspiration cytology
D trucut biopsy
E assessment for BRCA1 and 2 mutations with sentinel node biopsy

13. The MOST likely diagnosis is

A breast carcinoma
B fibrocystic disease
C fibroadenoma
D benign mammary dysplasia
E lipoma

14. A 20-year-old female is referred for recurrent epistaxis and bruising. She takes no medication. On examination she has no facial rash or lymphadenopathy. Her spleen is just palpable, and she has generalised bruising but no bone or joint tenderness. Immediate blood test results are

White cell count	$5 \times 10^9/L$
Hb	10 g/dL
Platelets	$25 \times 10^9/L$
ESR	55 mm/hr
MCV	90 fl
MCH	30 pg
MCHC	34 g/dL
Prolonged bleeding time	
Serum urea	6 mmol/L

The next MOST useful investigation would be

A bone marrow aspirate
B haemoglobin electrophoresis
C platelet autoantibodies
D Factor VIII:C and Factor VIII: vWF assays
E platelet aggregation studies

15. The MOST likely diagnosis is

A thrombotic thrombocytopaenic purpura
B idiopathic thrombocytopaenic purpura
C aplastic anaemia
D SLE
E von Willebrand's disease

16. A 70-year-old man presents with bruising and bone and joint pain. On examination he has nail splinter haemorrhages. The back of his legs are covered with haemorrhages into the muscles and ecchymoses. X-ray of his legs shows subperiosteal haemorrhages. The MOST likely diagnosis is

A idiopathic thrombocytopaenic purpura
B scurvy
C subacute bacterial endocarditis
D aplastic anaemia
E Henoch–Schönlein purpura

17. A 22-year-old female is noted to have both microcyctic and macro-cytic anaemia. She gives a history of intermittent diarrhoea. The MOST likely diagnosis is

A cystic fibrosis
B irritable bowel syndrome
C coeliac disease
D Crohn's disease
E ulcerative colitis

18. A 20-year-old healthy man presents with acute shortness of breath, fullness in the head and blackouts. He smokes 10 cigarettes a day and drinks socially. He is noted to have a ruddy plethora, JVP 6 cm and dilatation of veins on his chest wall. The MOST likely diagnosis is

A bronchial carcinoma
B Hodgkin's lymphoma
C non-Hodgkin's lymphoma
D cor pulmonale
E polycythaemia rubra vera

19. A 20-year-old homosexual man presents with proctalgia and bloody anal discharge. The MOST likely organism would be

A human papilloma virus
B chlamydia trachomatis
C neisseria gonorrhoea
D haemophilus ducreyi
E treponema pallidum

20. A 45-year-old man on lithium for bipolar disorder is started on ben-drofluazide for recently diagnosed hypertension. The MOST likely complication is

A decrease in efficacy of lithium
B none as there is no drug interaction
C lithium toxicity
D decrease in efficacy of thiazide
E increased sensitivity to thiazide

21. Heroin withdrawal may be distinguished from cocaine intoxication by which ONE of the following findings?

A pupillary dilation
B hypertension
C sweating
D vomiting
E fever

22. A 36-year-old woman diagnosed with premature ovarian failure now presents with bone pain. Her serum calcium, phosphate and alkaline phosphatase and urinary calcium are all normal. Recommended treatment for this patient may include all of the following EXCEPT

A bisphosphonate
B conjugated oestrogen (premarin)
C raloxifene
D conjugated oestrogen and norgestrel (prempak)
E calcitonin

23. The following statements regarding calcium are correct EXCEPT

A Calcium and sodium bicarbonate solutions may be administered simultaneously via the same route.
B The initial dose in a patient with tetany is 10 ml of 10% calcium chloride.
C Calcium is not suitable for tracheal administration.
D It is indicated for pulseless electrical activity caused by hyperkalaemia.
E Calcium may precipitate arrhythmias.

24. The following statements regarding fluoxetine are correct EXCEPT

A It is a selective serotonin reuptake inhibitor.
B It is indicated for premenstrual tension.
C It is indicated for bipolar disorder.
D It is indicated for obsessive-compulsive disorder.
E It has some antimuscarinic effects.

25. Which one of the following antiviral drug is LEAST advisable in pregnancy?

A efavirenz
B nelfinavir
C zidovudine
D didanosine
E nevirapine

26. A 20-year-old woman presents with fatigue, nausea, vomiting, and abdominal colic. She has been feeling unwell for many months now living as a squatter in a derelict old house. On examination she is noted to have signs of peripheral neuropathy with a wrist drop. Blood film shows basophilic stippling of red blood cells. The MOST likely diagnosis is

A thalassaemia
B iron poisoning
C lead poisoning
D Crohn's disease
E carbon monoxide poisoning

27. Which one of the following illicit drugs is still detectable in urine for up to 25 days since last used?

A cocaine
B cannabis
C methadone
D heroin
E amphetamine

28. The following are associated with Reiter's syndrome EXCEPT

A keratoderma blenorrhagica
B seropositive polyarticular, asymmetrical arthritis
C painful uveitis
D aortic incompetence
E circinate balanitis

29. A 40-year-old man presents with painful asymmetrical deforming arthritis involving the distal interphalangeal joints and lower back pain. His fingernails are pitted, with onycholysis and linear melanonychia. The MOST likely diagnosis is

A rheumatoid arthritis
B ankylosing spondylitis
C psoriatic arthritis
D osteoarthritis
E inflammatory bowel disease (IBD)

30. A 40-year-old woman presents with fever, symmetrical polyarthralgia affecting the fingers, wrists and knees and weight loss. She is also noted to have alopecia, oral and nasal mucosal ulceration. Her full blood count shows anaemia with thrombocytopaenia and raised ESR. The MOST definitive investigation is

  A rheumatoid factor
  B ANA
  C anticentromere antibodies
  D antibodies to double-stranded DNA
  E c-ANCA

31. A 50-year-old woman presents to medical outpatients complaining of pain and stiffness in the joints of her hands, worse in the mornings. The pain lasts for a couple of hours in the morning. On examination she has ulnar deviation, wasting of the small muscles of her hands, nail pitting and a rash on her knees. There is symmetrical involvement of the distal interphalangeal joints and metacarpophalangeal joints. The MOST likely diagnosis is

  A rheumatoid arthritis
  B psoriatic arthropathy
  C dermatomyositis
  D SLE
  E osteoarthritis

32. A 20-year-old man presents with morning back stiffness. He has a history of iritis. On examination he has an early-diastolic murmur. Chest x-ray shows bilateral diffuse reticulonodular shadowing. The MOST likely diagnosis is

  A Reiter's syndrome
  B Crohn's disease
  C rheumatoid arthritis
  D ankylosing spondylitis
  E sarcoidosis

33. A previously well 55-year-old man presents within 12 hours of the onset of chest pain suggestive of myocardial infarction. His ECG shows ST segment elevation greater than 0.2 mV in two adjacent chest leads. The MOST appropriate management would be

  A thrombolytic therapy
  B IV glycoprotein IIb/ IIIa inhibitor in addition to aspirin and unfractionated heparin
  C coronary angiography
  D percutaneous transluminal coronary angioplasty
  E coronary artery bypass graft

34. A 60-year-old man with a history of angina presents with chest pain. His ECG shows ventricular tachycardia. His pulse rate is 200/min, and his BP 80/50. Oxygen is applied by face mask. The FIRST action should be

    A administer sedation and call urgently for the anaesthetist
    B immediate synchronised cardioversion at 100J
    C immediate unsynchronised DC cardioversion at 200J
    D IV adenosine
    E IV lignocaine

35. A 70-year-old man collapses on the ward. His ECG shows ventricular fibrillation. He has a cardiac pacemaker. The minimum distance away from the pacemaker unit for placement of the defibrillator electrodes should be

    A 2 cm
    B 5 cm
    C 8 cm
    D 10 cm
    E 12 cm

36. Pulseless electrical activity in a cardiac arrest may be associated with all of the following EXCEPT

    A tamponade
    B thrombo-embolism
    C malignant hyperpyrexia
    D hypokalaemia
    E ruptured aortic aneurysm

37. A 60-year-old man complains of chest pain. His 12-lead ECG shows dominant R waves and ST depression in V1-V3. The lesion is MOST likely in the

    A left anterior descending coronary artery (LAD)
    B diagonal branch of the LAD
    C circumflex artery
    D right coronary artery
    E obtuse marginal branch of the LAD

38. The MOST appropriate management for this patient following oxygen, aspirin, GTN and morphine is

    A coronary angiography
    B percutaneous transluminal coronary angioplasty (PTCA)
    C coronary artery bypass graft
    D thrombolytic therapy
    E glycoprotein IIb/ IIIa inhibitor and non-fractionated heparin

39. A 50-year-old woman complains of episodes of diplopia and vertigo, worse after exercise. On examination the BP in her right arm is 120/80 and the BP in her left arm is 100/60. A left cervical bruit is noted. The most likely diagnosis is

A coarctation of the aorta
B transient ischaemic attack
C Takayasu's arteritis
D subclavian steal syndrome
E vertebrobasilar insufficiency

40. A 70-year-old man presents with nausea, vomiting and weakness. He has marked peripheral oedema. His medications include digoxin and chlorthalidone for congestive heart failure. Frusemide is administered to which he has marked diuresis of 10 litres and promptly collapses. His ECG shows prolonged P-R interval, inverted T waves and depressed ST segments. The MOST useful blood test is

A CK-MB and troponin
B serum urea and electrolytes
C digoxin level
D serum osmolality
E random cortisol

41. A 65-year-old woman presents to Casualty with breathlessness and chest pain. On examination her pulse is irregularly irregular and ECG confirms atrial fibrillation at a rate of approximately 180/min. You administer oxygen and gain IV access. The next most appropriate management would be

A heparin and warfarin anticoagulation
B immediate heparin and synchronised DC shock at 100J
C amiodarone 300 mg IV over 1 hr
D IV digoxin
E flecainide 100 mg IV over 30 mins

42. A 60-year-old man is admitted with congestive heart failure. JVP is 5 cm. His admission bloods are

White cell count	7×10^9/L
Hb	11 g/dL
Platelets	50×10^9/L
MCV	110 fl
MCH	31 pg
MCHC	34 g/dL
AST	45 IU/L (5–35 IU/L)
ALT	50 IU/L (5–35 IU/L)
GGT	190 IU/L (11–51 IU/L)
LDH	300 IU/L (70–250 IU/L)
Alk phos	300 IU/L (30–300 IU/L)
Serum glucose	5 mmol/L

The MOST likely cause of his congestive heart failure is

A folate deficiency
B vitamin B_{12} deficiency
C haemochromatosis
D alcoholism
E haemolytic anaemia

43. A 20-year-old man complains of high fever, rigors, productive cough with rusty-coloured sputum and pleuritic chest pain. On chest examination he has increased tactile fremitus and dullness to percussion in the right lower lung field. The MOST likely diagnosis is

A lobar pneumonia
B bronchopneumonia
C aspiration pneumonia
D pleural effusion
E lung abscess

44. The drug of first choice is

A cefotaxime
B tetracycline
C erythromycin
D flucloxacillin
E penicillin

45. A 25-year-old woman presents to Casualty with light-headedness and breathlessness. She complains of tingling and numbness of her hands. Arterial blood gas

pH	7.55
PaCO₂	3 kPa
PaO₂	14 kPa
H+	25 nmol/L
HCO₃	20 mmol/L

The MOST likely diagnosis is

A psychogenic hyperventilation
B salicylate intoxication
C pulmonary oedema
D tension pneumothorax
E pulmonary embolism

46. A 50-year-old obese man presents with headache and drowsiness. He has a history of snoring. He has warm extremities, a flapping tremor and a bounding pulse. On fundoscopic examination papilloedema is present. The MOST appropriate treatment would be

A flumazenil
B doxapram
C naloxone
D hyperbaric oxygen
E diazepam

47. A 50-year-old man presents with dysphagia. On examination he has increased jaw jerk reflex, fasciculation and wasting of the tongue, fasciculation and wasting of the small muscles of the hands and exaggerated lower limb reflexes. No sensory changes are present. The MOST likely diagnosis is

A Parkinson's disease
B multiple sclerosis
C myasthenia gravis
D amyotrophic lateral sclerosis
E pseudobulbar palsy

48. A 50-year-old man presents with progressive dementia over 6 months. His wife states that he is extremely forgetful. He drinks in moderation and smokes 20 cigarettes a day. He takes oxybutinin for urinary incontinence. On neurological examination he has lower extremity spasticity and extensor plantar responses with an ataxic gait. The MOST likely diagnosis is

A thiamine deficiency
B normal pressure hydrocephalus
C Friedreich's ataxia
D Alzheimer's disease
E Huntington's chorea

49. A 60-year-old woman with rheumatoid arthritis presents with neck pain and numbness and tingling in the thumb and first 2 fingers of the right hand. It is worse at night. On examination there is sensory loss in the right hand involving the lateral half of the ring finger and dorsal tips of the first two fingers. The patient is able to flex the inter-phalangeal joint of the index finger on clasping the hands (Ochner's test). The MOST likely diagnosis is

A complete median nerve lesion
B carpal tunnel syndrome
C median and ulnar nerve palsy
D cervical spondylosis
E cervical rib

50. The MOST useful investigation is

A lateral and antero-posterior cervical-spine x-ray
B MRI scan of the neck
C nerve conduction studies
D hand x-ray
E chest x-ray

51. A 30-year-old female presents with severe headache and vomiting. She is sensitive to light and also complains of neck pain. BP is 170/110 and pulse 50. On examination she has bilateral ptosis, dilated pupils and eyes are positioned down and out. On fundo-scopic examination bilateral papilloedema is present. Protein and glucose are present in her urine. Her mental status deteriorates rapidly. The MOST likely diagnosis is

A intracranial tumour
B subdural haematoma
C subarachnoid haemorrhage
D extradural haematoma
E intracerebral haemorrhage

52. Anorexia nervosa may be associated with all of the following EXCEPT

   A low white cell count
   B low haemoglobin
   C low urea
   D low bicarbonate
   E low potassium

53. A 70-year-old man presents to Casualty after falling when drunk. He complains of sudden numbness and tingling all over both his legs. He also complains of pain between the shoulder blades. On examination he has weakness in his lower extremities, hyperreflexia, positive Babinski, and clonus. The MOST likely diagnosis is

   A motor neurone disease
   B subacute combined degeneration of the cord
   C spinal cord compression
   D cauda equina compression
   E anterior spinal artery thrombosis

54. A 60-year-old man presents to Casualty with fever and neck pain on passively moving the chin towards the chest. Lumbar puncture shows

white cells	3000/mm³ predominantly neutrophils
red blood cells	1/ mm³
glucose	1.5 mmol/L (Blood glucose emmol/L)
protein	5 g/L

   The MOST likely organism is

   A mycobacterium tuberculosis
   B neisseria meningitidis
   C haemophilus influenzae
   D listeria monocytogenes
   E streptococcus pneumoniae

55. A 20-year-old male suffers from ataxia and dysarthria progressing over the past 3 years. On examination he has loss of position sense, lower limb weakness, extensor plantars and absent deep tendon reflexes. He is also noted to have a pes cavus deformity. The MOST likely diagnosis is

   A Friedreich's ataxia
   B motor neurone disease
   C multiple sclerosis
   D taboparesis
   E peroneal muscular atrophy (Charcot–Marie–Tooth disease)

56. A 40-year-old man presents with diplopia and pain over the left eye. His medication includes lisinopril and humulin insulin. On examination he has an almost total loss of eye movements but with sparing of lateral and downward eye movement on the left. His pupils are symmetrical, reactive to light and are of normal size and shape. The MOST likely diagnosis is

A complete III and IV nerve palsy
B mononeuritis involving the III nerve
C complete III nerve palsy
D complete III, IV and VI nerve palsy
E myasthenia gravis

57. A 30-year-old man presents with a right red painful eye. He complains of watering of the eyes and sensitivity to light. He has a history of recurrent cold sores. The most useful investigation is

A slit-lamp examination
B fluorescein dye test
C litmus paper for pH
D Schirmer's test
E smear for Gram-stain

58. A 45-year-old myopic woman comes to Casualty complaining of headache. She states that she also sees flashing lights and cannot see the lower part of objects on the right. Her vision is obscured by what is described as looking through murky water. On examination a field defect is confirmed. The MOST likely diagnosis is

A acute closed angle glaucoma
B uveitis
C migraine with focal aura
D transient ischaemic attack
E retinal detachment

59. A 60-year-old woman presents with sudden painless loss of vision in her right eye. There is no perception of light and there is an afferent pupillary defect. The retina is white with a cherry red spot at the macula. The optic disc is swollen. She is a known hypertensive. The MOST likely diagnosis is

A retinal detachment
B optic neuritis
C central retinal vein occlusion
D ischaemic optic neuropathy
E central retinal artery occlusion

60. A 70-year-old long-sighted woman presented to Casualty at midnight with vomiting that began three hours earlier and slightly worsening vision. The eyeball fells very hard on palpation. The conjunctiva is injected. The MOST likely diagnosis is

A acute angle-closure glaucoma
B anterior uveitis
C choroidiris
D retinal vein thrombosis
E temporal (giant cell) arteritis

61. A 40-year-old woman is referred for psychological assessment. Her latest preoccupation is with the size of her nose, which she believes is too large for her face. She spends several hours a day in front of a mirror. She has had several cosmetic operations to her face, but believes she is still unattractive. On examination her nose looks fine. She is MOST likely suffering from

A dissociative disorder
B obsessive compulsive disorder
C Munchhausen's syndrome
D body dysmorphic disorder
E somatisation disorder

62. Suicide rates are the highest among patients with

A schizophrenia
B alcoholism
C drug addiction
D borderline personality disorder
E major affective disorder

63. A 50-year-old obese man is brought to Casualty in a confused state. On examination he has nystagmus and is unable to move the eyes fully laterally. He walks with a broad-based gait. He is unaware of his surroundings and grows restless. The MOST likely diagnosis is

A subdural haematoma
B Creutzfeldt–Jakob syndrome
C Wernicke's encephalopathy
D Korsakoff's psychosis
E hypoglycaemia

64. An asymptomatic 60-year-old man is found to have an isolated raised alkaline phosphatase on routine biochemistry. His serum calcium and phosphate levels are normal. The MOST likely diagnosis is

A osteomalacia
B multiple myeloma
C Paget's disease
D liver metastases
E hyperparathyroidism

65. The incubation period for hepatitis B is

A 14–42 days
B 14–90 days
C 28–180 days
D 42–180 days
E 90–180 days

66. A 62-year-old woman who has recently undergone liver transplantation for primary biliary cirrhosis presents with pruritis and right upper quadrant tenderness. She has light-coloured stools and dark urine. Her amylase, bilirubin, uric acid, gamma-glutamyl transferase, transaminases are all elevated. Her alkaline phosphatase is 2000 IU/L (30–300 IU/L). The MOST useful initial investigation is

A abdominal ultrasound
B percutaneous cholangiogram
C ERCP
D liver biopsy
E abdominal CT scan

67. A 35-year-old female presents with anorexia, fever, abdominal pain, arthralgia and increasing jaundice. She also mentions that she has not had a period for several months. On examination she has acne, hirsuties, bruises, cutaneous striae, hepatosplenomegaly and jaundice. Her serum bilirubin, globulin and aminotransferases are high. The MOST likely diagnosis is

A primary biliary cirrhosis
B alcoholic Cushing's syndrome
C Wilson's disease
D acute viral hepatitis
E autoimmune chronic active hepatitis

68. An 80-year-old woman presents with dysphagia and weight loss. She complains of a sensation of a lump in her throat, bad breath, and regurgitation of undigested food. She has a history of recurrent chest infections. She does not smoke or drink alcohol. Physical examination reveals a low BMI and a visible lump on the left side of her neck, which is difficult to define on palpation. The MOST likely diagnosis is

    A squamous cell carcinoma of the oesophagus
    B pharyngeal pouch
    C achalasia
    D cricopharyngeal spasm
    E post-cricoid carcinoma

69. An 80-year-old man presents with a 2-month history of weakness, dark stools and worsening constipation alternating with episodes of diarrhoea. He has lost a stone in weight. He has a history of diverticular disease and has had 2 myocardial infarctions. Blood tests reveal anaemia, hyponatraemia, hypokalaemia and hypochloraemia. The stool is positive for occult blood. The most likely diagnosis is

    A left-sided colonic carcinoma
    B right-sided colonic carcinoma
    C ischaemic colitis
    D diverticulitis
    E gastric carcinoma

70. A 28-year-old Jamaican woman presents with acute onset of nausea, vomiting, epigastric pain and ascites. She does not take any medication apart from traditional herbal remedies. On examination she has tender hepatomegaly and profound ascites but no signs of heart failure. She has abnormal liver function tests. The ascitic fluid has high protein content. The investigation of CHOICE is

    A isotope scanning of the liver
    B hepatic venography
    C liver biopsy
    D ultrasound scan
    E abdominal x-ray

71. The MOST likely diagnosis is

    A primary biliary cirrhosis
    B hepatic vein thrombosis
    C alcoholic hepatitis
    D portal vein thrombosis
    E Meig's syndrome

72. A 50-year-old woman presents with an abdominal mass and back pain. She denies abdominal pain or abnormal vaginal bleeding having had her last period 9 months ago. Cervical smears have never been abnormal. On examination there is a central mass palpable to above the level of the umbilicus. On pelvic examination there is a palpable right adnexal mass. Urine HCG is negative. The MOST useful investigation is

A plain abdominal and lumbar spine x-rays
B CT scan of the abdomen and pelvis
C serum progesterone and β-HCG
D pelvic ultrasound
E CEA-125 tumour marker

73. A 65-year-old man presents with a 2-month history of vague lower abdominal pain, alternating diarrhoea with constipation and 4 kg weight loss. He has passed a small amount of dark red blood per rectum. There is anaemia. The MOST likely diagnosis is

A diverticular disease
B Crohn's disease
C ulcerative colitis
D angiodysplasia
E colorectal cancer

74. A 60-year-old man presents with sudden severe colicky pain and bloody diarrhoea that began after lunch 3 hours ago. He has a history of 2 myocardial infarctions. On examination: Temperature 39°C, BP 130/90, pulse 110/min regular. There is rebound tenderness in the lower left quadrant of his abdomen and there is fresh blood present in the rectum. There is a raised white cell count and mild anaemia. The MOST likely diagnosis is

A colon carcinoma
B diverticular disease
C inferior mesenteric artery ischaemia
D superior mesenteric artery thromboembolism
E Campylobacter infection

75. A 40-year-old woman presents with multiple symptoms. She states that for weeks she has felt tired with a loss of appetite. She has intermittent abdominal pain, diarrhoea and has lost half a stone in weight. On examination: temperature 36.5°C, supine BP 100/60 with a pulse of 90/min; postural hypotension, mild epigastric pain and a pigmented appendicectomy scar. The MOST likely diagnosis is

    A hypopituitarism
    B diabetes mellitus
    C Addison's disease
    D hyperthyroidism
    E Crohn's disease

76. A 25-year-old obese lady presents with mood swings, acne, secondary amenorrhoea and hirsutism. She has mild lower back pain, which she relates to her weight problem. She smokes 20 cigarettes a day and drinks alcohol at weekends. BP is 125/85 and urine dipstick is negative for glucose. The most likely diagnosis is

    A Cushing's syndrome
    B polycystic ovary syndrome
    C congenital adrenal hyperplasia
    D ovarian carcinoma
    E hypothyroidism

77. A 90-year-old man is noted to have a serum alkaline phosphatase of 1050 IU/L (30–300 IU/L) on routine blood tests. He is asymptomatic. His calcium, phosphate, and PTH levels are normal. The MOST appropriate management would be

    A nil
    B abdominal ultrasound scan
    C radionucleide bone scan of whole body
    D alkaline phosphatase isoenzyme fracionation
    E calcium carbonate 1.25 g/vitamin D^3 400 i.u. tablets b.d.

78. A 50-year-old man presents with loss of libido and gynaecomastia. His wife explains that he is always tired and moody. She states that he has physically changed from his holiday photographs. BP is 160/90 and urine dipstick is positive for glucose. The MOST useful investigation to establish the diagnosis is

    A thyroid function tests
    B short synacthen test
    C growth hormone
    D testicular ultrasound
    E oral glucose tolerance test

79. A 40-year-old woman presents with weight gain and depression. Her blood pressure is 150/90 and she has glycosuria. She complains also of secondary amenorrhoea and hirsutism. The most appropriate initial investigations would be

A 24-hour urine collection for urine-free cortisol assay
B overnight dexamethasone suppression test
C serum luteinising hormone and follicle stimulating hormone levels
D serum testosterone
E HbAIC

80. A 16-year-old male presents with gynaecomastia. On examination his arm span exceeds the trunk length and he has small, firm testes. The MOST likely diagnosis is

A testicular feminisation
B congenital adrenal hyperplasia
C Klinefelter's syndrome
D true hermaphroditism
E adrenal 5α-reductase deficiency

81. The following conditions are associated with short stature EXCEPT

A achondroplasia
B hypopituitarism
C rickets
D Crohn's disease
E Klinefelter's syndrome

82. A 45-year-old female who underwent mastectomy with axillary clearance 2 years ago now presents with excessive thirst and polyuria. Investigations show

Serum sodium	150 mmol/ L
Serum potassium	3.8 mmol/L
Serum calcium	2.8 mmol/L
Random serum glucose	9 mmol/L
Serum urea	6 mmol/L
Serum creatinine	100 μmol/L
Urine osmolality	150 mosm/kg

The MOST likely diagnosis is

A psychogenic polydipsia
B SIADH
C cranial diabetes insipidus
D metastatic breast cancer
E diabetes mellitus

83. A 50-year-old woman is noted to have a high serum calcium, low-normal phosphate and normal albumin on routine biochemistry test. She is asymptomatic. A subsequent serum parathyroid hormone (PTH) comes back as high. The MOST useful investigation to confirm the diagnosis is

A skull, hand, pelvis and chest X-rays
B ultrasound scan of neck
C radioisotope thallium/technetium subtraction scan of neck
D MRI scan of neck
E CT scan of neck

84. A 60-year-old man presents to Casualty drowsy and confused. Blood test results

Serum sodium	150 mmol/L
Serum potassium	5 mmol/L
Serum chloride	105 mmol/L
Serum bicarbonate	30 mmol/L
Serum urea	10 mmol/L
Serum glucose	40 mmol/L

The MOST likely diagnosis is

A hyperosmolar non-ketotic coma
B severe diabetic ketoacidosis
C meningitis
D encephalitis
E pre-renal renal failure

85. The following management is advisable EXCEPT

A 0.9% saline IVI
B heparin
C insulin at 3 U/h
D measure serum potassium hourly
E blood cultures

86. An 18-year-old known asthmatic presents with severe wheezing and a respiratory rate of 30 and a pulse of 120. She is using her accessory muscles and appears distressed. She is apyrexial. The most appropriate initial management would be

A IM adrenaline
B Oxygen and nebulised salbutamol
C IV dexamethasone
D Endrotracheal intubation
E IV pencillin

87. A 50-year-old man with insulin dependent diabetes mellitus presents with peripheral oedema and ascites. He has 3+ proteinuria. 24-hour urine collection contains 10 g of protein. His serum albumin is 15 g/L. The MOST effective initial management would be

A oral frusemide
B IV mannitol
C protein restriction
D increase fluid intake
E restrict salt

88. A 30-year-old woman presents with fever, cough, and haematuria. She had been in Egypt 2 weeks prior. On examination she has hepatomegaly. The MOST useful investigation to make the diagnosis is

A IV urogram
B urine for microscopy and culture
C KUB plain film
D cystoscopy
E renal and bladder ultrasound

89. A 35-year-old man presents with progressive weakness in his limbs over the past few days. He had a chest infection 2 weeks prior. On examination he has proximal muscle wasting, hypotonia and absent deep tendon reflexes. His lumbar puncture results are

Cells   4/cc lymphocytes
Chloride   110 mmol/L
Glucose   3.5 mmol/L
Protein   3 g/L

The MOST likely diagnosis is

A poliomyelitis
B botulism
C Guillan–Barre syndrome
D AIDS
E subacute combined degeneration of the cord

90. A 70-year-old man presents with confusion and urinary incontinence. He is pale; BP 160/100. On examination the bladder is palpable to the level of the umbilicus. Rectal examination confirms an
enlarged prostate. There is also peripheral oedema. Blood tests show

White cell count	7×10^9/L
Hb	8 g/dL
Platelets	100×10^9/L
Serum sodium	125 mmol/L
Serum potassium	6 mmol/L
Serum urea	60 mmol/L
Serum calcium	3.4 mmol/L

The working diagnosis is

A chronic renal failure
B acute renal failure
C benign prostatic hypertrophy
D prostate carcinoma
E myelomatosis

91. The MOST appropriate immediate step in management would be

A arrange urgent renal ultrasound
B slow bladder decompression with a sterile catheter
C measure 24 hour urinary protein and creatinine clearance
D arrange urgent IV urogram
E give 10 mls of 10% calcium gluconate and 15 units of insulin with 50
   g glucose 50% IV

92. The MOST appropriate treatment for moderate acne in an adoles-
cent female is

A erythromycin + topical keratolytic + cyproterone acetate for three
   months
B benzoyl peroxide 5–10%
C trimethoprim + erythromycin/benzoyl peroxide (Benzamycin)
D retinoic acid
E roaccutane

93. A 70-year-old woman presents with a lesion on her lower right leg,
which has been slowly getting larger over several months. There is a
single scaly flat non-tender red plaque 3×4 cm on the lateral side of
her lower leg. It is occasionally itchy. The MOST likely diagnosis is

A squamous cell carcinoma
B psoriasis
C melanoma
D Bowen's disease
E discoid eczema

94. A 20-year-old African female presents with tiny raised spots over her cheeks and neck. The papules are non-tender and non-pruritic but are multiple, scattered and unsightly. The MOST likely diagnosis is

A seborrhoeic warts
B dermatosis papulosa nigra (DPN)
C acne keloidalis nuchae
D molluscum contagiosum
E verruca plana

95. A 25-year-old man presents with an intensely pruritic rash over his hands, buttock and penis. The itching is worse at night. He had unprotected sexual intercourse a few days ago. On examination there are delicate scaling areas with threadlike linear tracks on the sides of his hands, palms and buttocks. His penis is covered with large, pruritic, crusted papules and nodules. The MOST likely diagnosis is

A crab lice
B scabies
C primary syphilis
D jiggers (tungiasis)
E Enterobius vermicularis (threadworm)

96. A 60-year-old Mediterranean woman presents with a month's history of rapidly progressive, generalised blistering eruption over her face, chest and axillae. On examination there are randomly scattered tense bullae associated with erosions and crusts. The blisters extend on digital pressure and are easily ruptured and weep. The MOST likely diagnosis is

A pemphigus vulgaris
B bullous pemphigoid
C bullous dermatitis herpetiformis
D erythema multiforme
E bullous impetigo

97. A 50-year-old woman, who is an avid sunbather, presents with a red forehead with a scaly rash. On examination the lesions multiple, discrete, small erythematous, with a keratotic surface and varying from a few millimetres to up to 1 cm in diameter; they are gritty to the touch. The MOST appropriate initial management would be

A photodynamic therapy
B metronidazole
C wide excision and graft
D topical flourouracil (efudix)
E intradermal triamcinolone

98. A 20-year-old woman presents with copious foul-smelling green vaginal discharge and sore throat. She last had unprotected oral and vaginal sexual intercourse 2 days ago. She is 3 months pregnant. The MOST appropriate management is

A take low vaginal swab for microscopy and culture
B take high vaginal swab for microscopy and culture
C take endocervical swab for virology
D take high vaginal, endocervical and pharyngeal swab for microscopy and culture and endocervical swab for virology
E take low vaginal, high vaginal and endocervical swabs for microscopy and culture and endocervical swab for virology

99. The MOST likely organism is

A chlamydia trachomatis
B trichomonas vaginalis
C neisseria gonorrhoea
D gardnerella vaginalis
E candidiasis

100. A 22-year-old female presents with frothy grey vaginal discharge. She states that she last had unprotected sexual intercourse 2 weeks ago. The vaginal discharge is noted to have a pH of 5 and emits a fishy odour on alkalinisation with potassium hydroxide. The MOST likely organism is

A neisseria gonorrhoea
B trichomonas vaginalis
C candidiasis
D chlamydia trachomatis
E gardnerella vaginalis

Answers to Paper Six BOFs

Criterion Referencing Marks

*   – 25–50% of candidates expected to get correct
**   – 50–75% of candidates expected to get correct
*** – 75–100% of candidates expected to get correct

The notional PASS MARK is 78%

1. B ***

2. B ***

3. E **

4. B ***

5. B *

6. A ***

7. C ***

8. A ***

9. A *** A serum K of <2.5 should be treated with IV potassium replacement. The local Public Health Doctor should be informed regarding a possible food poisoning outbreak from this restaurant.

10. E ***

11. A **

12. C ** FNA is less invasive than a trucut biopsy. FNA can also be used to distinguish between a cystic vs a solid lump.

13. C **

14. C ***

15. B ***

16. B ***

17. C ***

18. B *** In a fit young healthy man think of SVC obstruction as an emergency manifestation of Hodgkin's disease. The treatment is same day radiotherapy.

19. C ***

20. C **

21. E ** Fever is present with heroin withdrawal and not with cocaine intoxication.

22. B ** Unopposed oestrogen replacement puts the patient at unnecessary risk for endometrial carcinoma and is ill-advised. Prempak is a form of combined HRT and is a better choice. Raloxifene is licensed for the prevention of vertebral osteoporosis and is a selective oestrogen-receptor modulator.

23. A **

24. C ** Fluoxetine is contraindicated during the manic phase of bipolar disorder.

25. A *

26. C ***

27. B * Cannabis is detectable in urine for up to 27 days with chronic use and for years if a sample of hair is analysed.

28. B *** Reiter's syndrome is a seronegative polyarthritis.

29. C ***

30. D ***

31. B ***

32. D *** Ankylosing spondylitis is associated with both aortic regurgitation and pulmonary fibrosis. X-ray of the spine should show squaring of the vertebrae and a characteristic bamboo spine.

33. A ***

34. A *** The patient needs to be sedated prior to synchronised cardioversion and expert help is required.

35. E *

36. C *** PEA is associated with hypothermia and not hyperthermia.

37. D ** The ECG changes are consistent with a posterior MI.

38. D ***

39. D ***

40. B *** Digoxin toxicity may be precipitated by hypokalaemia. The ECG changes are consistent with hypokalaemia.

41. B ***

42. D *** The GGT is high and suggests alcoholism as the cause of the macrocytic anaemia and congestive heart failure.

43. A ***

44. E ***

45. A ***

46. B ***

47. D ***

48. B **

49. B **

50. C ***

51. C ***

52. D ** Anorexia is associated with a high bicarbonate level due to excessive vomiting.

53. C ***

54. E *** S. pneumonia meningitis is more common among the elderly.

55. A **

56. B *** This patient has a partial III palsy as the pupil is spared.

57. B *

58. E **

59. E ***

60. A *

61. D ***

62. E **

63. C ***

64. C ***

65. D ***

66. A ***

67. E **

68. B ***

69. A ***

70. C ***

71. B *** The patient has veno-occlusive disease secondary to bush tea (Jamaican herbal tea) containing pyrrolidizine alkaloids. This condition resembles Budd–Chiari syndrome.

72. D ** The mass is most likely an ovarian tumour.

73. E ***

74. C ***

75. C ***

76. B ***

77. A *** As the patient is asymptomatic, no treatment is advised at this time of his likely occult Paget's disease.

78. C ***

79. C ***

80. C ***

81. E ***

82. C ***

83. C *** This investigation is highly diagnostic for parathyroid adenomas and for pre-operative localisation of the parathyroid glands.

84. A *** The anion gap here is 20. Anion gap = (Na + K) − (Cl + HCO3).

85. A *** 0.45% saline should be used if the Na is >150.

86. C ***

87. A ***

88. B **

89. C ***

90. A ***

91. B ***

92. A **

93. D **

94. B *

95. B ***

96. A ** Nikolsky's sign is positive when the blisters extend on digital pressure.

97. D ** This is actinic keratosis.

98. D **

99. C ***

100. E **

Questions

1. Recognised complications of ulcerative colitis include

   A pyoderma gangrenosum
   B iritis
   C sclerosing cholangitis
   D ankylosing spondylitis
   E enterocolic fistula

2. Addison's disease is characterised by

   A postural hypotension
   B buccal pigmentation
   C menorrhagia
   D myalgia
   E constipation

3. Secondary amenorrhoea is associated with

   A uterine leiomyomata
   B thyrotoxicosis
   C endometriosis
   D menopause
   E anorexia nervosa

4. Clinical features of syndrome of inappropriate ADH (SIADH) include

   A peripheral oedema
   B higher urine than plasma osmolality
   C hypertension
   D normal renal function
   E hypokalaemia

5. Recognised causes of diabetes insipidus include

   A haemochromatosis
   B demeclocycline
   C postpartum pituitary infarction (Sheehan's syndrome)
   D lithium
   E histiocytosis X

6. Hashimoto's thyroiditis is associated with

A lymphadenopathy
B greater incidence in elderly men than women
C hyperthyroidism in the early stages
D firm and rubbery thyroid gland
E neutrophil infiltration of the thyroid gland

7. Pericardial rub may be heard in the following conditions

A Coxsackie virus infection
B Dressler's syndrome
C hyperthyroidism
D systemic lupus erythematosis (SLE)
E uraemia

8. Rapidly progressive proliferative glomerulonephritis is associated with

A extracapillary crescent formation in only few glomeruli
B Wegener's granulomatosis
C Goodpasture's syndrome
D Henoch–Schönlein purpura
E aspirin overdose

9. Recognised sexually-transmitted diseases include

A bacterial vaginosis
B condyloma accuminatum
C herpes simplex virus I
D moniliasis
E treponema pallidum

10. The following statements regarding atrioventricular block are correct

A Permanent pacing is required in all types of heart block after an acute anterior myocardial infarction.
B It may be caused by verapamil.
C It may be caused by adenosine.
D Wenckebach phenomenon has a high risk of sudden death.
E Stokes–Adams syndrome is associated with third degree AV block.

11. Causes of ptosis include

A lid xanthelasma
B myasthenia gravis
C third nerve palsy
D Grave's disease
E Pancoast's tumour

12. Hyperparathyroidism is associated with

    A depression
    B duodenal ulcer
    C polyuria
    D proximal myopathy
    E pseudogout

13. Recognised features of hypertensive retinopathy include

    A cotton wool exudates
    B microaneurysms
    C hard exudates
    D flame haemorrhages
    E comma-shaped conjunctival haemorrhages

14. Recognised causes of alopecia include

    A polycystic ovarian syndrome
    B iron deficiency
    C pernicious anaemia
    D Cushing's syndrome
    E tinea capitis

15. Recognised causes of leg ulceration include

    A syphilis
    B hereditary spherocytosis
    C Cryoglobulinaemia
    D necrobiosis lipoidica
    E neurofibromatosis

16. Sarcoidosis is associated with

    A iritis
    B finger clubbing
    C pyoderma gangrenosum
    D positive Mantoux test
    E hilar lymphadenopathy

17. The following statements regarding syphilis are correct

    A Aortic stenosis is common in tertiary syphilis.
    B Condyloma lata are a sign of primary syphilis.
    C Treponema pallidum crosses the placenta.
    D Secondary syphilis is associated with a generalised skin rash over the face, palms and soles.
    E Primary syphilis is associated with a painful hard chancre and tender regional lymphadenopathy.

18. The following statements regarding leptospira icterohaemorrhagica infection are correct

    A It is known as Weil's disease.
    B It is a spirochaetal infection.
    C During the immune phase, 10% present with meningism.
    D Presentation includes fever and myalgia.
    E Specific IgG leptospiral antibodies appear by the end of the first week.

19. Characteristic features of polycystic ovarian (PCO) disease include

    A hirsutism
    B acne
    C menorrhagia
    D infertility
    E obesity

20. Recognised features of endogenous depression compared with reactive depression include

    A early morning waking
    B auditory hallucinations
    C diurnal variation of mood
    D fleeting suicidal feelings
    E self-pity

21. Aortic dissection is a recognised complication of

    A Ehlers–Danlos syndrome
    B Marfan's syndrome
    C cystic medial necrosis
    D coarctation of the aorta
    E bicuspid aortic valve

22. A diagnosis of hypopituitarism would be supported by the following results

    A peak cortisol of 600 mmol/L (normal cortisol >550 mmol/L) on triple stimulation test
    B growth hormone of 15 mU/L (normal GH >20 mU/L) on triple stimulation test
    C TSH at 20 minutes of 15 mU/L (normal TSH at 20 mins – 3.9 to 30 mU/L) on triple stimulation test
    D microcytic anaemia
    E hypernatraemia

23. The following tumours commonly present in patients below 30 years of age

    A papillary carcinoma of the thyroid
    B non Hodgkin's lymphoma
    C teratoma
    D osteogenic sarcoma
    E cervical carcinoma

24. Hypocalcaemia is associated with

    A osteomalacia
    B sarcoidosis
    C Paget's disease
    D Addison's disease
    E renal osteodystrophy

25. Jaundice may occur with

    A Weil's disease
    B haemolytic anaemia
    C aspirin poisoning
    D chlorpromazine
    E infectious mononucleosis

26. Characteristic features of acromegaly include

    A carpal tunnel syndrome
    B diabetes insipidus
    C increased circulating growth hormone (GH) following bromocriptine
    D goitre
    E proximal muscle weakness

27. Depression is more common among

    A higher socio-economic groups
    B men than women
    C smokers than non-smokers
    D younger generation than middle-aged group
    E those with a physical disability

28. Paget's disease (osteitis deformans) is associated with

    A hypocalcaemia
    B normal bone turnover
    C severe bone pain alleviated by intravenous disodium pamidronate
    D pathological fractures
    E nerve deafness

29. The following drugs may be given safely at reduced doses in moderate to severe renal impairment

A atenolol
B co-amoxiclavulanic acid
C lithium
D trimethoprim
E warfarin

30. Recognised features of pharyngeal pouch include

A heartburn
B aspiration pneumonia
C halitosis
D hoarseness
E dysarthria

31. Falciparum malaria in endemic areas

A should be treated with intravenous quinine if unable to be taken orally
B should be treated with Maloprim (pyrimethamine and dapsone) as prophylaxis during early pregnancy
C can be prevented by chloroquine prophylaxis in coastal East Africa
D may be treated with oral quinine for 7 days followed by a stated dose of Fansidar (pyrimethamine and sulfadoxine)
E is the most common cause of benign malaria

32. Recognised treatment for supraventricular tachycardia include

A atropine
B verapamil
C adenosine
D flecainide
E lignocaine

33. Features of digoxin overdose include

A bradycardia
B tinnitus
C nausea
D hallucinations
E abdominal pain

34. In atrial fibrillation

    A digoxin is recommended in chronic atrial fibrillation
    B warfarin is advised in patients if the cause is mitral valve disease
    C in acute cases treat immediately with DC cardioversion prior to
       further investigations
    D warfarin is advised in patients with "lone" AF
    E in chronic AF the aim is control of ventricular rate

35. Features of autoimmune Addison's disease include

    A hyperkalaemia
    B hyperpigmentation of the palmar creases
    C hypocalcaemia
    D hypoglycaemia
    E abdominal pain

36. Achalasia of the cardia is associated with

    A gastro-oesophageal reflux
    B pre-malignancy
    C failure of relaxation of the cricopharyngeal sphincter
    D increase in ganglionic cells in the oesophageal myenteric plexus
    E recurrent pneumonia

37. Endometriosis causes

    A superficial dyspareunia
    B secondary dysmenorrhoea
    C intestinal stricture
    D external fistula formation
    E ovulatory pain

38. Clinical features of Turner's syndrome (gonadal dysgenesis) include

    A lymphoedema of the hands and feet
    B ambiguous genitalia
    C coarctation of the aorta
    D secondary amenorrhoea
    E absent breast development

39. Ectopic pregnancy may be associated with

    A serum β-human Chorionic Gonadotrophin (β-hCG) >6,000 IU/L
    B shoulder tip pain
    C per vagina (PV) prune juice spotting
    D salpingitis
    E the intrauterine contraceptive device (IUCD)

40. Secondary amenorrhoea is associated with

   A thyrotoxicosis
   B anorexia nervosa
   C polycystic ovarian disease
   D uterine leiomyomata
   E endometriosis

Answers to Bonus MCQS

Criterion Referencing Marks

* – 25–50% of candidates expected to get correct
** – 50–75% of candidates expected to get correct
*** – 75–100% of candidates expected to get correct

1. TTTTF **

2. TTFTF *** Addison's disease is also associated with diarrhoea and amenorrhoea.

3. FTFTT ** Secondary amenorrhoea is also associated with polycystic ovarian (PCO) disease, premature menopause and myxoedema.

4. FTFTF ***

5. FTTTT **

6. FFTTF ** Hashimoto's thyroiditis is more common in women aged 60–70 and is an autoimmune disorder associated with lymphocyte and plasma cell infiltration.

7. TTFTT **

8. FTTTF ** RPGN is associated with >60% extracapillary crescent formation. Aspirin is associated with tubulo-interstitial nephritis.

9. FTFFF *** Bacterial vaginosis is caused by gardnerella and is associated with excessive douching. Condyloma accuminatum is better known as genital warts. HPV 16 and 18 are associated with cervical cancer. HSV II and not I is associated with genital herpes. Monoliasis or candidiasis occurs in diabetics or immunocompromised individuals. Trepenoma pallidum is the organism that causes syphilis.

10. FTTFT ** Permanent pacing is recommended following Mobitz Type II and complete heart block. AV blockers include digoxin, verapamil, adenosine and β-blockers. Wenckebach phenomenon or Mobitz Type I is considered benign.

11. TTTFT *** Pancoast's tumour is associated with Horner's syndrome.

12. TTTFT ***

13. TFFTF *** Microaneurysms and hard exudates are signs of diabetic retinopathy. Comma-shaped conjunctival haemorrhages are seen in sickle cell disease.

14. TTTTF ** Alopecia may result from androgen excess in females.

15. TTTFF **

16. TFFFT *** Sarcoidosis is associated with a negative Matoux test and a positive Kveim test.

17. FFTFF *** Aortic regurgitation occurs in tertiary syphilis. Condyloma lata are a sign of secondary syphilis. Secondary syphilis is associated with an itchy maculopapular rash sparing the face. Primary syphilis is associated with a painless hard chancre arising 2–4 weeks post-exposure and painless regional lymphadenopathy.

18. TTFTF * 50% of patients will present with meningism in the immune phase. IgM leptospiral antibodies appear by the end of the first week.

19. TTFTT ***

20. FTTTT ***

21. FTTTF ***

22. FTFFF ** Hypopituitarism is associated with a normochromic normocytic anaemia and a dilutional hyponatraemia. The results of the triple stimulation test should show a GH <20 mU/L, peak cortisol <550 mmol/L and a TSH at 20 minutes of <3.9 mU/L.

23. TFTTF *** Hodgkin's lymphoma and not Non Hodgkin's lymphoma is associated with a younger presentation.

24. TFFTT ***

25. TTFTT ***

26. TFFTF ***

27. FFFFT **

28. FFTTT *** Bone turnover is increased.

29. TFTTF **

30. FTTTF *** Pharyngeal pouch is associated with dysphagia and not dysarthria.

31. TTFTF ** According to the BNF, chloroquine once weekly is recommended prophylaxis in North Africa and the Middle East. Elsewhere chloroquine is recommended in conjunction with proguanilice 200 mg daily. Doxycycline is recommended in chloroquine-resistant areas such as Oceania. Benign malaria is associated with Plasmodium vivax. The BNF lists advice centres that can be consulted.

32. FTTTF *** PSVT is treated with adenosine. Flecainide is used to treat SVT associated with Wolff–Parkinson–White syndrome. Lignocaine is used to treat VT and VF.

33. TFTTT ***

34. TTFFT *** In acute cases, the cause of AF should be managed first – alcohol toxicity, thyrotoxicosis, chest infection and the rhythm converted next. "Lone" AF (AF of unknown cause) does not require anticoagulation as the risk of emboli is very small.

35. TTFFT *** Addison's disease is associated with hypercalcaemia and buccal pigmentation. Disease associations include Grave's disease, Hashimoto's disease, IDDM, hypoparathyroidism, pernicious anaemia, and ovarian failure.

36. FTFFT *** Achalasia of the cardia is associated with failure of relaxation of the lower oesophageal sphincter and a decrease in ganglionic cells in the myenteric plexus.

37. FTTFT *** Endometriosis is associated with deep dyspareunia.

38. TFTFT ** Other clinical features include short stature, primary amenorrhoea, webbed neck, widely spaced nipples, horseshoe kidney and spontaneous fractures.

39. FTTTT ***

40. TTTFF **